CONTENTS

sm98008095
4/99
£18.00
HJH P
(Bar)

HEALTH PROMOTION AND HEALTH EDUCATION SERIES

Leo Barić

PEOPLE IN SETTINGS

Foreword by
Dr Ilona Kickbusch
WHO Geneva

Barns Publications

0951697366

Also by Leo Baric:

**Health Promotion and Health Education
CURRICULA FOR COURSES AND WORKSHOPS**

**Health Promotion and Health Education
PROBLEMS AND SOLUTIONS (OUT OF PRINT)**

**Health Promotion and Health Education
THE ORGANISATIONAL MODEL**

**Health Promotion and Health Education
EVALUATION, QUALITY, AUDIT**

**Health Promotion and Health Education
HANDBOOK FOR STUDENTS AND PRACTITIONERS**

*Copyright © Leo Baric
First Edition 1998*

ISBN 0 95 16973 6 6

*Published by Barns Publications, 14 High Elm Road, Hale Barns,
Altrincham, Cheshire, WA15 0HS (Fax 0161 980 7446, Tel 0161 980 8276)*

FOREWORD

Ilona Kickbusch PhD
Director
Division of Health Promotion, Education & Communication
WHO HQ
Geneva

The settings approach to health promotion and health education extended the activities from HP/HE experts to all the people in various settings (schools, hospitals, enterprises, communities, etc.). It is, therefore, a most appropriate time to publish a book for people in settings that promote health. This year marks the anniversaries of events, which have been important for the developments in this field. It is the 50th anniversary of WHO and on a more local level it is also the 50th anniversary of the National Health Service in the UK. It has also been 20 years since the Alma Ata Declaration and the commitment of member states to Health for All by the Year 2000, and over 11 years since the Ottawa Charter, which has had such a profound impact on the practice of health promotion and health education. It was in Ottawa that the foundations were laid for the shift of emphasis from diseases and health threats (the medical model) to people with health problems who live, work and play in different settings (the organisational model). Looking back over the past 11 years, it is encouraging to establish that the change has been justified and is now widely accepted throughout the world.

The Ottawa Charter (1986) affirmed the importance of healthy living and working conditions, as well as peace, shelter, education, food and income as essential prerequisites for health. This was followed by the Adelaide Recommendations (1988), which emphasised the importance of a healthy public policy for the health of a nation. The next international conference was held in Sundsvall (1991) and provided an opportunity for bringing together people with shared interests in public health, environment and ecology. It recognised the prime importance of a sustainable environment as a necessary condition for health of a population. The latest international conference in Jakarta (1997) produced The Jakarta Declaration, which deals with "New Players for a New Era - Leading Health Promotion into the 21st Century". After reaffirming the commitments undertaken during previous international conferences, it lists the following priorities for health promotion in the 21st century:

- Promote social responsibility for health;
- Increase investments for health development;
- Consolidate and expand partnerships for health;
- Increase community capacity and empower the individual; and
- Secure an infrastructure for health promotion.

Anniversaries usually provide opportunities for taking stock of what has been happening in the past and for mapping out the future. The Jakarta Conference did both and called on WHO to provide the leadership and support to build a global health promotion alliance.

The settings approach was fully confirmed by the Jakarta Declaration. The challenge now is to envisage taking the setting approach to a new level of organizational development and practical application. One of the main postulates of the Ottawa Charter, the enabling role of various formal health promotion and health education institutions, will require theoretical underpinning and the inclusion into teaching programmes on different levels. There is still a lot of work to be done in supporting the arguments that "health is an asset" in economic terms and that "health is a worth-while investment", as well as further developing the mechanisms for production and distribution of health promotion and health education as parts of the health service industry.

It is possible to envisage a future where quality driven health promotion and health education will be a part of local, national as well as international programmes and activities. To this end the present efforts invested in the development of specific health promotion and health education standards and specifications for activities within different settings is the best indicator of future changes.

This latest book by Leo Baric represents a continuation of his efforts to build a theoretical framework for health promotion and, following his previous publications in this field, brings health promotion to a practical level of application. It is aimed at people engaged in integrating HP/HE into various settings or in creating health promoting settings, and who will not have had the opportunity of reading more elaborate descriptions in Baric's previous books.

The book addresses the need of practitioners of various professional and occupational backgrounds for a practical handbook in which they can find the necessary information about "how to do it in the field". In addition to providing the reader with an opportunity to revise the basic knowledge about methods of defining the problems and choosing the appropriate solutions, it takes the concept of a "health promoting setting" to its logical conclusion: a "health promoting setting" should consist of "health promoting parts" with all its implications. It also provides the reader with an insight into health promoting settings and how to go about initiating them and helping in their creation and operation. It also makes a contribution to the understanding of the setting approach, by differentiating between the activities on an administrative and a consumer level within a setting.

The last section of the book deals with accountability within a quality-driven health promotion and health education. Whereas evaluation has been appropriate for problem based interventions, the general accountability of people involved in health promotion and health education in settings requires a wider approach: assessments of the setting, evaluation of interventions, external audit, and where appropriate, quality assessment of the processes and outcomes.

The future, however, seems to indicate that the direction of new developments will be in the area of quality management as a permanent and continuous process. The author suggests a special variation of quality management, adjusted to the needs of health promotion and health education, which would utilise standards, which have been specifically developed for health promoting settings and are linked to a generally recognised accreditation process. In this way, health promotion would introduce a culture of continuous monitoring and assessment and provide a feedback, including participatory processes for all stakeholders of the setting instead of evaluation, which is usually, if at all, carried out at the end of the programme or project. Contributions such as Baric's in this book, together with some other recent publications, indicate the 'coming of age' of health promotion.

Chapter 1

PRESENT SITUATION

Introduction
The organizational model
Settings as organizations
People in organizations
Future issues

Changes in the practice of health promotion and health education (HP/HE) are the result of the historical developments which have had profound effects, first on health education and later on health promotion. The most important events marking these changes may be considered on the international and the UK level.

International developments

The activity known today as 'health education and health promotion' has a pre-history as well as a history. The transmission of experience necessary for survival has enabled the human race to survive and improve living conditions. More recently this experience has been transmitted in an increasingly structured way, through collecting knowledge and institutionalizing the practices relevant to survival, among which health is one of the most important.

Fifty years ago, the creation of the World Health Organization as part of the United Nations, provided the international mechanism for the systematic collection, validation and development of experience relevant to survival and the improvement of the quality of life. The transmission of this experience was the responsibility of health education, an activity subsequently differentiated into health education and health promotion. WHO mechanisms for the development of both activities include World Conferences. These have publicized their findings in a number of resolutions, charters, declarations and reports.

A brief summary of these conferences (see diagram p.11) includes the main watersheds that have been responsible for bringing HP/HE to the present stage.

Alma Ata (1978)

Numerous developments in conceptualizing health and in the delivery of health care followed the Declaration emerging from the 1978 Alma Ata Conference, of which only most important are listed:

- Health is considered to be the basic human right, a principle that took certain aspects of health care out of the hands of the medical profession and made it a topic for politicians and the legal profession;

- Inequities in health among the population groups and regions are not acceptable and the concept of 'health for all' was adopted;

- There was a differentiation between the fields of activities of health education and health promotion, the former being concerned with the individual or group influences based on the concepts of competence and equity and the latter with environmental influences including physical and social environment together with individual's adjustment to these influences.

The Ottawa Conference (1986)

The First International Conference on Health Promotion met in Ottawa in 1986. It was strongly influenced by the contributors from Toronto, who produced a paper 'Toronto 2000', which declared it to be a 'Healthy City'. From this starting point, the idea of healthy cities as special settings originated. This concept was later extended to other settings.

The conference produced a charter for action to achieve 'Health for All by the Year 2000' and beyond. Although the Ottawa Charter is a comprehensive document, for our purposes it will be sufficient to mention its two main contributions to the future practice of health promotion:

- the outline of a methodology, which includes the tasks of *enabling, mediating and advocating* as the means of helping people to maintain and improve their health within the framework of a 'healthy public policy' and the creation of 'supportive environments';

- the change of emphasis from health problems to *people with health problems in settings*, which broadens the area of activity from a restricted health care system to a larger system of various settings (family, school, hospital, enterprise, and so on).

The conference was a response to growing expectations for a *new public health* movement in the light of the needs of industrialized countries, as well as other regions of the world. Health promotion action involves building a healthy public policy, creating supportive environments, strengthening community action, developing personal skills and reorienting health services.

The Adelaide Conference (1988)

The Second International Conference on Health Promotion was held in Adelaide in 1988. It was concerned with the development of *healthy public policies*. The conference ended with a set of Recommendations, which defined the strategy for healthy public policy action.

The Recommendations defined 'healthy public policy' *as being concerned with health and equity in all areas of policy including the accountability for the policy impact on health.* The main aim of healthy public policy is to create a supportive environment, which will enable people to lead healthy lives. It is a cross-sectoral endeavour to create a health-enhancing social and physical environment and to allow people to make easier healthy choices, reflected in their lifestyle. The value of health as an asset has been redefined to link economic, social and health policies into an integrated action characterized by equity, easy access and positive developments.

The Recommendations defined the following specific areas for action: supporting the health of women; food and nutrition; tobacco and alcohol; creating supportive environments; developing new health alliances; and the commitment to global public health.

The Sundsvall Conference (1991)

The Third International Conference on Health Promotion was held in 1991 in Sundsvall, Sweden. The main topic of the conference was the creation of *supportive environments* for health.

The conference produced a 'Statement', which issued a call to action for everyone to participate in creating a supportive environment, which should be taken up by all communities, countries and governments. A part of the supportive environment deals *with inequities and problems of poverty, as well as access to essential health care.* One of the main issues raised at the conference was the achievement of global accountability for maintaining a health-supportive environment.

The Jakarta Conference (1997)

The latest international conference in Jakarta (1997) produced the Jakarta Declaration, which deals with 'New Players for a New Era - Leading Health Promotion into the 21st Century'. After reaffirming the commitments undertaken during previous international conferences, it lists the following priorities for health promotion in the 21st century:

- Promoting social responsibility for health;
- Increasing investments for health development;
- Consolidating and expand partnerships for health;
- Increasing community capacity and empowering the individual;
- Securing an infrastructure for health promotion.

The Present Situation

The settings approach, introduced by the Ottawa Charter, was fully confirmed by the Jakarta Declaration. The challenge now is to envisage taking the settings approach to a new level of organisational development and practical application. One of the main postulates of the Ottawa Charter, the importance of the enabling role of people in various institutions, active in health promotion and health education, emphasises the need for the development of a theoretical underpinning and its subsequent inclusion into teaching programmes on different levels. There is still much work to be done in supporting the arguments that 'health is an asset' in economic terms or that 'health is a worth-while investment', as well as further development of the theory underlying the mechanisms for the production and distribution of health promotion and health education as parts of the health service industry.

Events following the Ottawa Charter (Baric, 1994, Appendix 1), created a situation in which HP/HE was faced with a completely new ball game, with new stakeholders and new players, where rules have been changed and even the goal posts have been moved. There are very few skills that can be carried over from the old game, to be used in the new game. We need to explore how HP/HE can adjust to this new situation. The changes include the differentiation between health promotion and health education, the shift of emphasis from the medical problems people have or are at risk from (the 'blame the victim' approach), to a focus on the people themselves, experiencing medical problems, while living, working and playing in different settings. This change of emphasis to people and their health, demands that attention should be paid to environmental factors (settings within a specific social and physical environment), as well as personal factors (life style, genetic inheritance, competence, motivation, adjustment to the environment) associated with people's health. HP/HE is gradually adjusting to these changes by using an organisational approach, and addressing people's socioculturally influenced life style in addition to their individual behaviour or actions. The consequences of this adjustment include the recognition that:

- the environment in which people live, work and play includes both a physical as well as social environment;
- settings are organisations with specific structures (including the distribution of power), which have specific functions and are of different scales;
- in settings, there are varied partners with specific languages and cultures (stakeholders, management, employees, customers);
- partners have specific agendas, including activities which can be health-related or health directed;
- health-directed activities can take the form of health promotion in a setting or of a 'health promoting setting';
- instead of a paternalistic approach *("what should we do for them?")*, the shift emphasises an enabling participative approach *("what can they do for themselves and how can we help?")*.
- assessment of a setting requires a comprehensive approach, this goes beyond the traditional evaluation of specific interventions and includes the concept of general accountability, which could in the future take on the form of 'quality type' continuous assessment.

It is, therefore, necessary to revise the issues related to the organisational approach and to place the settings within that framework, which include:

- recognition of the differences in approach between health promotion and health education as means of enabling people to deal with the threats to their own health, mediating between the consumers and providers of health care and advocating for the rights of the consumers;
- readjusting the approaches to new partners in different settings, taking into account their specific agendas, language and mechanisms as a part of an organisational model;
- giving up the idea of health promotion and health education as excluding the work of HP/HE professions and developing a multi-sectoral approach with people in various settings carrying out health promotion and health education activities as a part of their regular tasks and using their professional responsibilities according to their specific status;
- introducing where appropriate the concept of a 'health promoting setting' with all the relevant implications;
- extending the concept of evaluation to include the assessment of the setting as well as impact assessment, the evaluation of interventions, quality assessment of the processes and products, and measuring the achievements by using as indicators the health gain of the consumers;

This is the present situation in which health promotion and health education operate, and anyone active in this field should be aware of the issues mentioned if they aspire to interact with others working in this field. This overall picture is summarised in the following diagram:

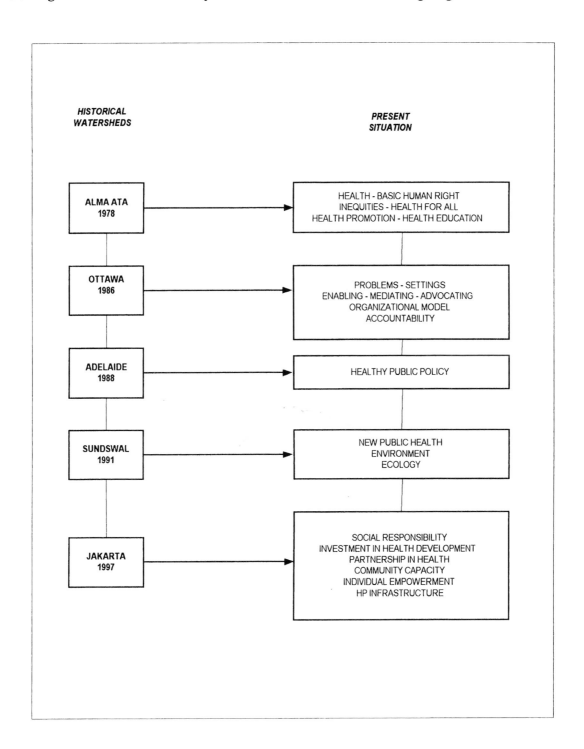

UK Developments

With the change in the UK government in 1997, new policies and strategies for the provision of health care within a modern and dependable health service have emerged. These have been described in the Government White Paper *The New NHS* (1997) and a Government Green Paper *Our Healthier Nation* (1998). This section deals only with issues raised in the latter document, that are relevant for HP/HE.

Public Health

The document discusses Public Health within the framework of a *Contract for Health*. This contractual approach, if it is to be beneficial for the health of the population, requires further development in terms of specifications, defining the rights and duties of both parties entering such a contract.

The Green Paper should be commended for emphasizing the need for a *'health impact assessment'* (3.11 p.32). This approach should not only ensure positive outcomes for the consumers but should also look at the wider consequences of such an approach. The advantage of a health impact assessment lies in providing an opportunity for the use of a simulation model to discover the various possible outcomes, without actually carrying out the program only to find possible errors and negative outcomes. It must be assumed that the health impact assessment will precede the implementation of policy, following the lines of other existing types of assessments, such as Environmental Impact Assessment, Technology Impact Assessment and social impact assessment.

Within the 'new approach to Public Health' (3.5 p.29), the emphasis is on the need for research (3.19 p.30), including scientific assessment and public perception (3.21 p.30), and the ability of people to use the information (3.23 p.30). A suggestion is made about the methods of achieving these aims (3.24 p.30/31). The document is nevertheless not clear about the topics of research and it would be prudent to make *a clear statement about striking a balance between research into problems and research into and testing of solutions.* A lesson should be drawn from the mistakes of the previous government's health policy, which included incorporating health promotion within the GP contract. After spending two years and £200 million it was found that there was no difference in the state of health between patients who were exposed to this kind of health promotion and those who were not ('Daily Telegraph', 19/7/93 p.16). The reason is very simple: nobody specified how the GPs should go about meeting the set targets. The health promotion and health education methods involved were taken for granted and were based on a 'common-sense' cognitive model of telling people what is good for them and expecting them to follow the advice, which practitioners of HP/HE know does not work. There is a great deal of evidence about the different abilities of people to understand information and use it, as well as about the different mechanisms involved in decision-making by different population groups. There is also a danger that the new approach to Public Health, of which health promotion and health education are an action aspect, will not address this problem and thus will not avoid the mistake made by the previous government.

To avoid this error, greater emphasis should be given to the study of solutions, including health promotion and health education approaches. Medical science studies medical problems and the pharmacological industry studies, tests and provides relevant solutions. A similar approach to health promotion and health education solutions would require sufficient resources and strict standards, based on tested methods, which could ensure that the accountability currently applied to medical interventions is matched by the accountability of agents who are involved in enabling people to make appropriate decisions and to undertake necessary actions with regard to their health.

Problems and Settings

The Green Paper takes good account of the most recent developments in health promotion and health education, as recommended by WHO, including the shift of emphasis from medical problems (the medical model) to people with medical problems, who live, work and play in different settings (the organisational model). The document lists (3.71 p.48) a number of priority problems (heart disease and stroke, accidents, cancers and mental health), as well as a number of problems of local significance (asthma and respiratory diseases, teenage pregnancy, infant mortality, backpain, rheumatism and arthritis, diabetes and oral health). The document also lists a number of settings (school, work-place, and neighborhood) to which other very important settings could be added, such as the health care system, the family and other special groups. The document also states that the government will continue to work with WHO on the European and global levels (3.16 p.33). From this, it can be assumed that the government accepts the Ottawa Charter, which, among other aspects, recommends the appropriate methods of intervention (enabling, mediating, advocating).

The following list of problems and settings should help in a systematic planning of relevant interventions.

When planning an intervention the first step should be to examine every problem according to the setting in which the intervention takes place. This can be illustrated by an example in which the various recommendations are summarized in a matrix, so that the planners can explore their inter-relationships. As already mentioned, appropriate aspects of HP/HE planning are:

Priority problems	Heart disease and stroke, Accidents, Cancers and Mental health
Local problems	Asthma and respiratory disease Teenage pregnancy Infant mortality Backpain Rheumatism and arthritis Diabetes Oral health

	Settings
Settings	School
	Workplace
	Neighbourhood
	(Health care system, family, etc)
Approaches	Socio-economic
	Environmental
	Life-style
	Services
Methods	Enabling
	Mediating
	Advocating

Using a matrix approach, illustrated in the following set of tables, helps to focus the understanding of the interrelated issues in various approaches.

Table 1: Problems and settings

PROBLEMS	SETTINGS			ADDITIONAL SETTINGS		
	SCHOOL	WORK-PLACE	NEIGHBOUR-HOOD	HEALTH CARE	FAMILY	SPECIAL GROUPS
HEART DISEASE & STROKE						
ACCIDENTS						
CANCERS						
MENTAL HEALTH						
Asthma & Respiratory Diseases						
Teenage Pregnancy						
Infant mortality						
Backpain, Rheumatism, Arthritis						
Diabetes						
Oral health						

For example, if we take one of the settings mentioned (school), then this can be explored according to the approaches recommended in the document (socio-economic, environmental, lifestyle and services). Each of these approaches will have specific requirements in dealing with different health problems. Any intervention will need to be very precise in describing each approach for each disease or an approach appropriate to a combination of several diseases at one time.

Table 2: EXAMPLE :HEALTHY SCHOOL - Problems and approaches

PROBLEMS	APPROACHES			
	SOCIO-ECONOMIC	ENVIRONMENTAL	LIFESTYLE	SERVICES
HEART DISEASE & STROKE				
ACCIDENTS				
CANCERS				
MENTAL HEALTH				
Asthma & Respiratory Diseases				
Teenage Pregnancy				
Infant mortality				
Backpain, Rheumatism, Arthritis				
Diabetes				
Oral health				

(A similar matrix will be required for each setting)

If the matrix method is adopted, then each approach for each health problem needs to be described in terms of the most appropriate health promotion and health education methods, defined in the Ottawa Charter as 'enabling, mediating and advocating'. If we now take the school as the chosen setting, and the socio-economic approach, it is possible to explore each method in relation to each of the problems mentioned in the Green Paper.

This procedure can be further refined by using one of the methods (enabling), and examining how it can be related to the relevant aims, objectives, indicators and criteria for this method according to each of the health problems.

Table 3: HEALTHY SCHOOL – Socio-economic approach : Problems and methods

PROBLEMS	SOCIO-ECONOMIC APPROACH			
	ENABLE	MEDIATE	ADVOCATE	EVALUATION QUALITY, AUDIT
HEART DISEASE & STROKE				
ACCIDENTS				
CANCERS				
MENTAL HEALTH				
Asthma & Respiratory Diseases				
Teenage Pregnancy				
Infant mortality				
Backpain, Rheumatism, Arthritis				
Diabetes				
Oral health				

In this way it is possible to develop a systematic approach for each problem within each setting, considering each approach, each method and the required definition of aims, objectives, indicators and criteria. This successfully satisfies the preconditions necessary for meeting the requirements for accountability, by means of assessment, evaluation, quality control and the measurement of outcomes in terms of the health gain of consumers.

Table 4: HEALTHY SCHOOL – Socio-economic approach : Problems and the method of enabling

PROBLEMS	METHOD OF ENABLING			
	AIMS	OBJECTIVES	INDICATORS	CRITERIA
HEART DISEASE & STROKE				
ACCIDENTS				
CANCERS				
MENTAL HEALTH				
Asthma & Respiratory Diseases				
Teenage Pregnancy				
Infant mortality				
Backpain, Rheumatism, Arthritis				
Diabetes				
Oral health				

Table 4 shows how one of the methods (enabling) can in turn be related to the relevant aims, objectives, indicators and criteria for this method, with respect to each of the health problems. In this way it is possible to develop a systematic approach for each problem within each setting, considering each approach, each method and the required definition of aims, objectives, indicators and criteria

The matrix approach helps to develop the understanding of interrelated issues in approaches. The implementation of Green Paper proposals would require similar matrices for each of the elements mentioned. Planners will need to decide which of the elements of these matrices is being implemented and will need to work out the details for their intervention.

Health promotion and health education within certain settings have a long tradition. For example, there is a long-standing tradition of health promotion in schools, general practices, hospitals, enterprises etc. Nevertheless, they have only been used as catchment areas for approaching a specific population group such as pupils, patients and the workforce. New developments arise from the introduction of the concept of a 'setting' as an organizational framework for planning the activity, taking into account all the mechanisms and processes which characterize a setting. This represents a qualitative difference from traditional health promotion *in* a setting. As a further elaboration of this approach, the introduction of the concept of a 'health promoting setting' adds a new dimension to the planning process. It requires a change in the organizational climate, in the establishing of organizational goals and the introduction of participative management practices. The outcome of this new approach has been the development of an appropriate organizational model within which the activity of health promotion and health education needs to be planned and carried out (Baric, 1994).

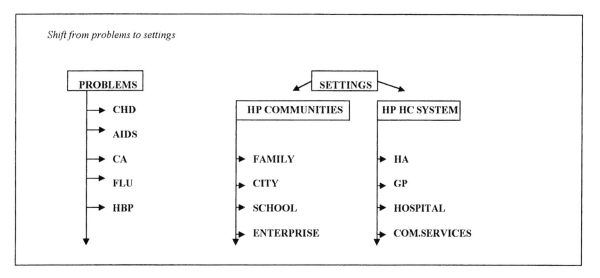

The focus on people in settings has enlarged the number of agents who are expected to be active in health promotion and health education as a part of their daily roles within the community. They now include parents, local politicians, teachers, employers and others, and within the health care system, medical and paramedical professionals as well as managers. In practice, the various settings operate by introducing internal changes and externally by creating *networks* and *alliances*.

The idea of networking is very important in the context of the methods of assessment now prevalent in many settings, which deal with the quality of procedures and outcomes in a production process. Networks can be established between similar settings, such as schools networks or organizational networks.

The concept of alliance refers to a formal relationship between settings of a different kind (e.g. a school and a hospital). It provides the opportunity for reducing potential conflicts and developing co-operation between different types of settings where the members are engaged in the similar task of improving their health.

Example of networks and alliances

ALLIANCES	NETWORKS		
Hospital 1	Hospital 2	Hospital 3	Hospital n
School 1	School 2	School 3	School n
Enterprise 1	Enterprise 2	Enterprise 3	Enterprise n
Etc.	Etc.	Etc.	Etc.

The developments in Europe arising from the emphasis on the settings approach have resulted in the re-thinking of existing practices. The new demands required a change in the theoretical background, in the type of agents involved and in the methodology of change, which has led to the change of emphasis from a medical to an *organizational* model. This model encompasses the structures and the functions of organizations or settings and provides a theoretical background for the understanding of individual activities within such settings as organizations. A consequence of this innovation has been the need for people engaged in health promotion and health education to become acquainted with organizational theory, as well as with the set of values and language used by the members of such organizations.

Defining the New Concept

The application of the new focus on health promotion in settings will depend on the ability of those concerned to understand the difference between health promotion ***in a setting*** and ***a health-promoting setting:***

- Health promotion in a setting has a long tradition and implies the introduction of health promotion and health education interventions (programmes, projects) into a specific setting;

- A health promoting setting is a new concept, which implies a change in the policy and strategy of a setting by including health promotion and health education aspects into the daily activities, a full participation of all the components of that setting, and the introduction of the assessment of health promotion and health education or its inclusion into the existing quality assessment system of that setting.

The inclusion of most of the members within a setting in health promotion activities requires a wider definition than usual of the role of health promotion 'agents'. The rapid increase in the body of knowledge and empirical case studies relevant to the practice of health promotion has resulted in the development of a theoretical basis for the activities and the empirically backed methods of defining the problems and solving them. The redefinition of the role of people engaged in health promotion can be achieved by:

- **Revising the curricula** concerning the teaching of the subject matter of health promotion and striking a balance between the theories related to organizations and management, medical topics, and health promotion approaches and methods (Baric, 1995b). This can be achieved by encouraging intervention studies, which will enable all professional groups within a setting to work out their needs according to the aims of their work as well as the best learning methods according to their expectations; it will involve consultations with the existing teachers of the subject matter; it will require preparation of new teaching material; it will require the adjustment of qualifications to the needs of various professions and occupations; and it will be necessary to develop a theoretical base for teaching this extended curricula on an academic level.

- The newly revised curricula will depend on the **definition of the 'educational product'**. For this, it will be necessary to explore the potential health promotion aspects of many professional and occupational roles and redefine them in that light. This can be achieved by allowing members of various professions and occupations to explore their own capabilities and needs within the planned intervention studies in various settings; by discussions and agreement with educational institutions offering various professional qualifications and in-service training programmes, to integrate health promotion into their existing curricula; and by reaching agreement on shared standards for qualifications in health promotion.

- The concept of **accountability** needs to be introduced into health promotion activities, together with the appropriate auditing. This can be achieved by defining the settings approach as a 'people-based' approach, and examining people's rights and duties related to health matters; by using assessment and simulations as a tool in planning interventions; by including into auditing the possible negative, as well as positive outcomes; by accepting the new concept of 'green auditing' and applying it to health promotion interventions; by organizing expert committees, workshops, seminars and meetings of a multi-professional and multi-occupational nature to discuss these issues; by publicising the behavioural norms concerning health promotion activities, as well as sanctions for the deviants; and by using existing or developing new mechanisms for the assessment of health promotion within the framework of quality management.

SETTINGS AS ORGANIZATIONS

The settings in which people live, work and play can be of different kinds and different levels of complexity, from a nuclear family to an international corporation or a national army. All these settings can be defined as organizations, each of which *represents a social entity, recognised by its structure and functions.* A health promotion and health education intervention using a setting's approach should, therefore, take into account relevant aspects of the study of organizations.

There are many definitions of an organization, most of which agree in principle but differ in the emphasis given to various components. For example, Robbins (1990) states: *"an organization is a consciously co-ordinated social entity, with a relatively identifiable boundary, that functions on a relatively continuous basis to achieve a common goal or set of goals".* In other words, an organization represents a group of people (social entity), who consciously co-ordinate their activities (management) for the achievement of common goals (function) on a more or less permanent basis. It is characterised by a set boundary, which defines who is a member of that organization and who is not. The relationship between members is defined by implicit or explicit contracts (norms), which represent the structure of that organization.

The *structure* of an organization is composed of statuses/roles associated with the goals (*function*) of that organization. Status denotes a position within a structure, whereas a role denotes the performance of the incumbent of a status. In other words, status and role are two aspects of the same thing. The structure and the function jointly represent the 'character' of an organization. Depending on the type of an organization, the structure will manifest different degrees of complexity represented by the number and arrangement of statuses/roles. It will involve different levels of formalisation of these statuses/roles, and it will differ in the degree of centralisation or decentralisation of power in that organization. There are two main types of organizational structure: the vertical and the horizontal. A *vertical* organizational structure is more common and represents a model of 'top management', 'middle management' and the executive or work force. The *horizontal* model aims at simplifying the channels of communication by reducing the number of people in top management, excluding middle management where possible, emphasising the importance of the work force and allowing for a more direct contact between the decision makers and the decision executors.

The distribution of *statuses/roles* represents the 'design' of an organization, which undergoes constant changes according to the new demands and conditions affecting the achievement of its goals. It is a well known fact that the most common method of solving an organizational problem is by means of 'reorganization' or changes in the design, which may provide personal satisfaction to the management, and a feeling that something has been done about the problem without necessarily solving the problem.

Organizations are a part of and operate within a world that is constantly changing. This implies that to survive and be successful, organizations must either be in a position to control the outside world or to adjust to the necessary changes (March & Simon, 1958). A common approach to organizational change is based on a cognitive model of decision-making, which does not always apply in real life. The model of organizations as open systems seems to be more appropriate. Change within such a model depends on a number of *'imperatives'* in the management of change (Dawson, 1992), which include: elements of rationality and irrationality; relationship between decision and action; variable participation in decision and action from people in different position in the structure; and processes of learning and creativity.

Change effected in an organization can usually be traced to a felt *'need'* by its members, which can be based on rational or irrational arguments. The rational arguments may be associated with the changes in the environment (market, technology, product image, etc.), whereas the irrational arguments usually reflect the wishes of the change agents who may believe that an organizational change may solve the internal problems facing the organization.

There is, however, no doubt that the survival of an organization will depend on its *adaptive powers* to meet the new situations. This is the area of interest of numerous 'organizational development' theories and practices (Clark and Krone, 1972) which have resulted in a variety of programmes addressing the topics of communication, problem-solving, decision-making and conflict resolution.

More recent work on changes in organizations is associated with the idea of organizational learning. The concept of a *'learning organization'* (Pascale, 1990) treats organizations as open systems and is based on the assumption that, like individuals, organizations can also learn. Organizations can be thought of as using the 'experiential learning method' and thus learn by doing, through experimenting and adjusting, using a feed-back mechanism that provides the management with indications about the outcomes of introduced changes. Schien (1985) advocates a 'double loop learning' method, which, in contrast to the single loop learning method, is open to outside influences, involves participation of all members and encourages creativity. Once the importance of the organizational potential to learn has been recognised, a number of different learning approaches can be developed. The emphasis now is on open-minded, creative learning management styles.

In the light of the 'health promoting setting' approach, there is a need to rethink the necessary organizational changes. Existing forms of organizational change might be sufficient in a setting where people intend to start some HP/HE activities, such as for example, to introduce the HP/HE subject matter into a school curriculum. The creation of a health promoting setting will, however, require more fundamental and radical changes in structure, role definitions and the culture of the organization. This need has been recognised by management experts, who devise new labels for radical new ways of managing change and coping with the restructuring of organizations. One such approach deals with the need to *'reengineer the setting'*. The idea of reengineering had a big impact in industry. It represents a new development in organizational change (Hammer &

Champy, 1993), and implies starting over instead of tinkering with the system or making incremental changes. *"Reengineering is the fundamental rethinking and radical redesign of business processes to achieve dramatic improvements in critical, contemporary measures of performance, such as cost, quality, service and speed"*. Hammer and Champy published their ideas in the form of a 'Manifesto for Business Revolution'. The key word in their definition is 'process'. They suggest that managers should concentrate on the process instead of the tasks, jobs, people and structures. This new approach was adopted by a number of large companies (IBM Credit, Ford Motor and Kodak) and seems to have produced some visible advantages and results. The process aims to meet contemporary demands of quality, service flexibility and low cost.

All of this is possible because of the growth and application of information technology, which is envisaged not only as an improvement in the existing ways of storing and retrieving information but as a revolution in utilizing information for creative thinking and the management of organizations for the purpose of creating preconditions for continuous change.

Organizational Goals

Other recent developments reflect the study of social and cultural changes in Europe defined as 'post-modernism'. Theorists of post-modernism challenged positivist conceptions and substituted interpretation for explanation. They have only just begun to turn their attention to organizations and available studies are limited although some of their general ideas have entered mainstream management theory (see Morgan, 1986, 1993).

This new conceptualisation builds on the work of Foucault (1977), Marcuse (1964), Habermas (1971), Derrida (1976) and Moi (1985). All approaches agree, however, that the main purpose of an organization is to achieve some defined goals. Therefore, the concept of 'organizational effectiveness' is considered to be the main concern of any organization theory and a part of any study of organizations. In operationalising this concept, it is clear that the definition of 'effectiveness' will depend on the indicators and criteria used. Researchers have used different approaches in the study of effectiveness, but overall they can be described in terms of four main approaches (Cameron, 1984):

- *Goal attainment*. The indicator is the level of attainment of the set goals, which requires specific and well defined goals that are measurable.

- *Systems approach*. The indicators are related to the processes associated with the acquisition of inputs, processing and producing outputs presupposing a causal relationship between inputs and outputs.

- *Strategic constituencies approach*. The indicator is the level of satisfaction of expectations of those constituencies in the environment on which an organization depends for support and existence.

25

- *Competing values approach.* This relates the various indicators to three models: the human relations model (emphasis on a cohesive and skilled workforce); the systems model (emphasis on flexibility and ability to acquire resources); and the rational-goal model (emphasises the need for existence of specific plans and goals and high productivity and efficiency).

Since the choice of indicators and criteria will vary according to the individual who carries out the evaluation of an organization, it is clear that the definition of 'effectiveness' is subjective, although most definitions will include goal achievement, maintenance of the life cycle of the organization and a successful relationship with the environment in which it operates and on which it is dependent. These would be part of an answer to the question whether an organization is effective or not.

As we have seen organizations are systems in which people perform to achieve a certain purpose or goal. The exploration of people's actions in organizational situations is known as the study of *organizational behaviour.* The term is here being used in the strict sense, concentrating on individuals and their behaviour. Sometimes management theorists use the term loosely, to refer to organization theory, structure and function as well. The difference is between behaviour in organization and behaviour of organizations.

Organizational behaviour involves some psychological concepts, relating to perception, motivation, learning and personality. It also includes concepts from social psychology, relating to groups, their formation, structure, social control and effectiveness. An important area included is the study of the impact that technology has on individuals working lives. Another broad area includes the study of management, decision-making, conflicts and the distribution of power.

For the purposes of this part, it will be convenient to differentiate between two aspects of organizational behaviour, the perspective of management and the perspective of the workforce.

The Management Perspective

The relationship between the structure and the management of an organization has been the topic of many studies, resulting in a number of schools of thought and theories.

Theories and Approaches

The first writers in the field of management have been subsequently labeled as protagonists of the so called '*classical management theory*' (Pugh, 1991) The writings of a number of people prominent in the management of various successful organizations and enterprises used their experiences as guidelines or suggestions for others to follow.

In the study of behaviour in organizations two strands are discernible: the behavioural sciences approach and the management sciences approach. The first draws on the theories and methods of *behavioural sciences.* Early developments used a traditional behavioural science approach (Berelson and Steiner, 1964), adopting a positivist, scientific approach to the study of human behaviour in organizations, employing empirical evidence collected in a 'scientific' way.

This approach was supplemented by the qualitative descriptive approach of Elton Mayo (1945), whose work on the 'Hawthorne effect' led to the human relations' movement in industry. The observations of workers in the Hawthorne plant showed that attention to human needs, no matter what form it took, improved productivity. This highlighted the human aspect of the workplace. This was followed by a number of other writers who extended the idea of 'industrial humanism' to other situations. Another important contributor was Rogers (1942), who developed insights important for organization theory and management practice through his client-oriented therapy and counseling methods. Moreno (1953) contributed to the study of organizations through his sociometric method of analysing human relationships within groups. Lewin (1935) with his field theory and group dynamics also provided a basis for understanding of organizations as groups.

The accumulation of studies in this field and the use of the *operational research* methods gradually brought about the recognition of a special field of organizational development, which also included *human resources management*. The latter was initially concerned with the two main tasks of managers: productivity and the quality of work life.

The opening of markets in the 1980s and the inclusion of partners from the Far East changed the rules of the game insofar that the existing strict descriptions of the organization design had to be modified. The new approach sometimes known as the *'contingency approach'*, which had been developed in the 1960s, and which succeeded the classical management theory and the human relations theories, was faced with the task of meeting these new needs. The general idea underlying this new approach was the recognition of the fact that people carry out work within certain environments, including cultural environments, and that the adjustment of people to that environment will be contingent on the prevailing circumstances. Hunt (1979, p.189) states: *'contingency theory refers to attempts to understand the multivariate relationships between components of organizations and to designing structures piece-by-piece, as best fits the components. This approach rejects earlier theories of universal models for designing formal structures and argues that each situation must be analysed separately'*.

Management as an Activity

The second development affecting the study of people in organizations is *management theory*. Management in general refers to the activity of people exercising authority over the activities and performances of other people. In a formal sense, management is carried out within a structured organizational setting, directed towards achieving aims and objectives through the efforts of other people, using specific systems and procedures (Mullins, 1992).

Being a manager may be interpreted as performing a certain *function* or as occupying a certain *status*. These are very general interpretations, which can often be overlapping and are interchangeable.

There is also often confusion over the meaning of 'management' as compared to 'administration'. In fact in some languages management is translated as administration (French). The term 'management' is now widely accepted while 'administration' is interpreted as a part of the management process.

The common *activities* of management include planning, organizing, command, coordination and control. Another interpretation of management treats it as a social process, which includes judgement and decision in determining plans and in using data to control performance; and guidance, integration, motivation and supervision of the personnel carrying out the operations.

There are many definitions of the *tasks and contributions* of managers, which involve most of the concepts mentioned earlier. They can be summarised as: setting objectives, ensuring that they are carried out by means of motivation and development of human resources, and controlling the outcomes. A good description of the concept of 'manager' was given by Brown (1974), who describes the manager as a person who has more work than he can do himself and has to delegate some of it to others, for whom he is accountable to higher authorities.

Another recent development in the manager's role is *just-in-time* planning, which refers to obtaining stocks of raw materials and parts necessary for production, where lengthy warehousing is replaced by the delivery of materials and parts just when they are need. This reduces capital investment and forces the producer to establish long-term relationship with the provider of raw materials or parts.

An important aspect of the manager's activity is concerned with *personnel* policy. This includes the selection and assessment of personnel, within a successful organizational structure, by defining the roles and securing optimal conditions for work. This role includes manpower planning and employment, salary and wage administration, education training and development, welfare, health and safety services and industrial relations.

Another managerial status is that of a line manager, who is in charge of a department or unit, generally responsible for the production process, essential for the achievement of the goals of the organization. Line managers are part of a complex management structure and have a clear role definition including power and accountability.

To be able to achieve relevant tasks a manager should, according to Mullins (1992), have the following *attributes*: technical competence, social and human skills including decision-making, and the ability to conceptualize problems and to see them in all their complexity.

Managerial Behaviour

The background to the study of the behaviour of a manager is derived from theories as a part of organizational behaviour and especially concerned with *motivation*. Motivation is reflected in the direction and persistence of action and explains why a person may continue with a particular course of action in the face of difficulties and problems. Mitchell (1982) describes four common characteristics, which underlie the definition of motivation: motivation is typified as an individual phenomenon; it is usually described as intentional; it is multifaceted and the purpose of motivational theories is to predict behaviour.

McGregor (1987) argues that there are basically two different managerial approaches, related to managers' attitudes towards people. **Theory X** is based on the traditional assumptions about organizations, which accepts the following generalizations: the average person is lazy and has an inherent dislike of work; most people must be coerced, controlled, directed and threatened with punishment if the organization is to achieve its objectives; and the average person avoids responsibility, prefers to be directed, lacks ambition and values security most of all. The central principle of Theory X is direction and control through a centralised system of organization and the exercise of authority. **Theory Y** is at the other extreme of the continuum. It is based on the central principle of integration of individual and organizational goals. It assumes that work is as natural as play or rest, and that people will exercise self-direction and self-control in the service of objectives to which they are committed; commitment to objectives is a function of rewards associated with their achievement; given the right conditions the average worker can learn to accept and to seek responsibility; the capacity for creativity in solving organizational problems is distributed widely in the population; and the intellectual potential of the average person is only partially utilised. Whereas in Theory X motivation occurs only at the physiological and security levels, in Theory Y, motivation is assumed to occur also at the affiliation, esteem and self-actualisation levels.

A third example is **Theory Z** exemplified by management style in the Japanese culture (Ouchi, 1984), which emphasises the need to manage people in such a way that they can work together more effectively. Theory Z management style includes: long-term employment, often for a life-time; relatively slow process of evaluation and promotion; development of company-specific skills and a moderately specialized career path; implicit, informal control mechanisms supported by explicit formal measures; participative decision-making by consensus; collective decision-making but individual ultimate responsibility; broad concern for the welfare of subordinates and co-workers as a natural part of a working relationship and informal relationships among people. The best known UK application of Theory Z has been in Marks & Spencer's (Tse, 1985).

Managerial Assessment

As one would expect, the crucial role of the manager(s) in an organization has attracted researchers from many disciplines. For our purpose, it is of interest to note the ways managers are assessed. Langford (1979) identifies four broad groups of indicators used in the studies of managerial effectiveness, which include:

- the manager's work - decision-making, problem solving, innovation, and management of time and handling information;

- the manager himself/herself - motivation, role perception, coping with stress, seniority and average salary grade for age;

- the manager's relationships with other people - subordinates, superiors, peers and clients; handling conflicts and leadership role;

- criterion of general effectiveness - allocation of resources, achieving purpose, goal attainment, planning, organizing, coordinating, controlling.

Within this general framework, a number of authors have developed various *instruments* for the assessment of managers, emphasising one or more of the mentioned areas of enquiry. Among the most quoted authors are Blake and Mouton (1985), who developed a Managerial Grid with two principal dimensions (concern for production and concern for people); Likert (1961), whose System 4 Management includes the principle of supportive relationships, group decision-making and high performance aspirations; Drucker (1968), who developed the Management by Objectives (MBO) approach, which is often used to describe a style of management which attempts to relate organizational goals to individual performance and development through the involvement of all levels of management. It includes the following principles: the setting of objectives and targets; participation by individual managers in agreeing about objectives and criteria of performance for each unit; and review and appraisal of results. Reddin (1970) developed a three-dimensional model of managerial behaviour, covering task orientation, relationship orientation and management style, as the combination of the two.

The Workforce Perspective

The study of people at work has been the concern of a wide range of scientific disciplines, including politics, economics, sociology and psychology. Each of these scientific disciplines has looked at the problems people meet at work from a different angle and developed models and theories to explain them. Whereas the study of management started from a wide range of premises and tended to converge to a recognised subject of management studies, the study of the workforce developed in exactly the opposite way. Starting from psychological interpretations such as motivation, it has diverged into a whole set of different models and theories. The contributing studies come from political sciences, economics, sociology, psychology, medical and management sciences.

Management Sciences

The management sciences have concentrated on the study of the performance of the workforce (Mitchell and Larson, 1987). The classical theorists believed that the difference in performance was associated with differences in workers' personality traits and abilities. Since this could not fully explain the differences in performance, behavioural scientists came up with the idea that personal satisfaction produces high performance even under most difficult conditions. They soon found out that even very satisfied workers could manifest variations in their productivity. This failure of explanation was followed by the assumption that future performance could be predicted on the basis of past performance. The outcome was that a worker with a good track record would be rewarded by promotion to a new position. An exaggeration of this assumption came to be called the 'Peter Principle' (Peter & Hall, 1969), which states that by applying this criterion to promotion means that people will be promoted until reaching the level of their incompetence, since without a good past performance no promotion should have taken place. The absurd conclusion from this assumption is that all the jobs (especially the top ones) are at present occupied by people who reached their level of incompetence since they have not been further promoted. Although this principle is very simplistic, it served to illustrate how unreliable an indicator past performance could be for future achievements.

The contingency approach to performance effectiveness postulates that it depends on the proper match between the worker and the job. The job of the management is to ensure that the right people are doing the right job under the right conditions. The outcome of such an approach has been the development of appropriate methods for the selection of personnel, based on an appropriate job analysis, and followed by an appropriate performance appraisal and reward system.

Job Analysis

If the idea is to match individuals to jobs, then it follows that it will be necessary to know precisely what the job is and what kind of demands it may put on the worker who is supposed to carry it out. The methods of job analysis vary, but usually depend on the collection of information by observation, statistical analysis of various measurements and by interviewing others who already perform that job. The job analysis forms the basis for the job description and should be used in assessing the applicants. This description is usually accurate in technical details but does not touch on the sensitive issues, which may differentiate a successful from a poor performer. To compensate for this shortcoming, researchers have been developing increasingly more sophisticated methods of measurement. This includes *professionally developed questionnaires*, which cover all the aspects considered to be relevant to job performance. Another research method uses the *critical incident technique*. Workers are asked to describe incidents, which lead to a good or a bad performance. The analysis of the answers provides a behavioural description of a good and a bad performer. On the basis of characteristics, which could include behaviour, skills, knowledge and abilities, it is believed possible to identify the attributes a successful applicant should have. It should be noted that such a job specification should not be allowed to fossilize, and should be regularly updated to include all the new developments associated with the organization and the expected performance. Carrying out a job analysis is, therefore, a skilled activity and requires certain knowledge and skill in collecting and analysing information. Special skills are required for making inferences on the basis of the information collected, useful in the next step, in personnel selection, which is the selection of candidates.

Candidate Assessment

This will depend on how successful the job description was, on the recognition of individual differences in personal characteristics of the applicants, and the selection of those, which are pertinent for the job performance. The methods of assessment of candidates include a number of approaches:

The most common is the *interview*, which is aimed at providing the employer and the candidate with a personal experience of learning as much as possible about each other. There are a number of different guidelines for conducting interviews and emphasizing various pertinent points, which should be included. More recently, the assessment of candidates has also included *psychological tests*. These can aim at assessing the candidate's mental abilities, muscular and motor coordination, personality traits and physical and sensory capacities. Job descriptions will define which of the tests are appropriate. As a result of the complexity of job requirements it is sometimes beneficial to use *assessment centers* for the selection of job applicants. Such an assessment center usually combines a whole variety of methods combined into an evaluation package. The information gathered can be used for selection, promotion, training and development of employees. An assessment center usually includes a number of professional assessors able to administer complex tests and other assessment tools, which is not usually available in a company or organization. The assessment usually takes 1-3 days and candidates' performance is rated by themselves, their peers, and the assessors. All this information is used to predict the future performance of a candidate. The increasing variety of assessment methods implies that not one of the existing ones is satisfactory. A new, recently developed approach, is the use of *work samples*, i.e. simulation of situations, which closely correspond to the actual work situation in which a candidate is tested and assessed. The main assessment judges whether the candidate's performance in a simulated exercise will accurately reflect the performance in a real life situation. For some jobs such as typists this has been a standard method of testing, whereas for some other jobs it has been dependent on the development of appropriate technology, such as flight simulators, etc. The most popular work sample technique for managers is known as an '*in-basket' test*. It includes placing the most characteristic items of a manager's job (memos, invoices, etc.) in an in-basket and asking the candidate to play the role of the manager and deal with this in-basket material.

In addition to various methods appropriate for the selection of candidates it may be necessary to provide the candidate with the possibility of a making realistic assessment of the job in question. The method developed for this purpose is *job preview*, which provides the candidate with all the necessary information about the job and an opportunity to become personally acquainted with other people working on the same or similar jobs in the company. This method has been shown to be very successful in allowing the candidate to develop a realistic picture of the job in question and is reflected in the low turnover of the workers participating in this process.

Performance Appraisal System

The assessment of the performance of employees depends on the precision of a job description, which should include the expectations concerning their performance, but also depends on the motivation of workers, associated with the existing reward system. Methods of assessment can take many different forms, the outcome of which will influence the administrative decision related to promotion, transfer, dismissal, wage and salary administration and bonus pay. Assessment will also be used as the indicator for various employee development programmes.

Appraisal techniques can include measures of *volume or quantity* of output, which can be assessed against preset standards associated with a specific job. They will include the assessment of *quality* as indicated by spoilage, rejected items, or any other indicator of failure; and can also include measures of *lost time,* through absenteeism or tardiness; and involvement in *training and promotion* can also be included if it is appropriate for a certain position. In jobs which do not have generally agreed upon standards of performance the assessment will have to be done on the basis of *subjective judgments* of supervisors or assessors. This subjective assessment can be based on some absolute standards or by comparison with other people.

The **instruments** for assessment are many and usually include a set of questions with the possibility of ranking the answers (i.e. from 'exceptionally good' to 'poor'). Instruments, which use absolute standards, are based on previous job assessments. They often include a *check list* of various behavioural patterns or actions which are then rated. These instruments can be more sophisticated by including weighted checklists and behaviourally anchored rating scales.

The **problems** associated with performance assessment are usually due to errors made by the raters or can occur due to single criterion problems instead of using all the relevant ones. Some errors arise from differences among jobs and among the raters.

Performance assessment is important not only for the employer but also for the employees. Through the mechanism of *feed-back*, the employees can be informed about their performance so that they can adjust. The outcomes of assessments suggests the need for counselling, additional training, addressing the problem of motivation, or the adjustment of some other environmental or behavioural factors. Most promising, however, is to allow the employees themselves to participate in the development of assessment instruments.

Since performance assessment is part of a more general *evaluation process*, it is necessary to consider the questions of who is doing the evaluation, how often it is carried out, its ethical and legal aspects, the recording of outcomes, and the consequences of such an evaluation. All these issues confront management and are very often a topic of interest for trade unions.

Systems of Reward

One of the main reasons for performance assessment is to provide information associated with the distribution of rewards or punishments. The *reward* mechanism is a very important aspect of the motivation of employees to fulfil expectations or even exceed them. The *punishment* aspect can operate positively or negatively, depending on the general situation in the organization, the situation on the job market in general and the form the punishment takes.

Most jobs include two types of rewards. The *intrinsic* rewards are considered to be a part of job performance and they are expressed in terms of personal satisfaction, feeling of competence, self-fulfillment etc. The *extrinsic* rewards are considered to be a part of the formal reward system and include pay increases, promotion and some other 'benefits', such as unemployment compensation, disability insurance, hospital benefits, private health and security benefits, retirement and life insurance, special employee services, meals and transportation, and compensation during vacations, sick leave, jury duty and lunch time. Most of these benefits, however, are not strictly limited to performance but are associated with specific position or type of job and serve as a general motivation for people occupying these positions. Only pay and promotion rewards are linked to performance and are distributed according to certain preset standards. In some organizations both the intrinsic and extrinsic rewards are in operation and, where they are not sufficient, a special system of bonus rewards is introduced. This bonus system is directly linked to performance.

The *problems* with a performance based reward system are mainly associated with the equity of the system, the level of aggregation at which performance is measured, salary versus bonuses, and the confidentiality of the pay and rewards.

These changes in emphasis are taking place at the time when we are facing two important watersheds, which will serve as incentives for producing long lasting and fundamental commitments in the field of health promotion and health education. The first one is the exciting prospect of planning future health promotion and health education activities for the new millennium with the start of the year 2000 and the second one of even greater practical importance is the celebration of the 50 years of the World Health Organization in the year 1998, when the new concepts and approaches for the next millennium will be formally set out. On an *organizational* level both occasions will provide opportunities for assessing the past achievements and planning new approaches, whereas on a *consumer* level these two occasions will provide an opportunity to remedy the past omissions and take the activities from the organizational to the consumer level.

If we want to improve on the past performances and take the health care system together with the supporting role of health promotion and health education, into the new millennium, it will be necessary to critically assess what has been achieved and even more so how it has been achieved and thus achieve improvements and avoid past omissions. If we do not want to continue with the perpetuation of the same mistakes in the next millennium, a critical assessment of the past performances will allow us to draw some conclusions as to the new measures to be taken in the near future. Although this critical assessment is an ongoing process, it is possible to already now suggest some improvements and corrections of our approaches.

'Scientific Rigour'

The multisectoral approach required that in addition to 'professional' health promotion and health education agents, other professions and occupations become active in this field. The lack of a rigorous scientific basis for health promotion and health education resulted in other professions rejecting this activity or inventing their own version of the activity. This has been reflected in the discussion about the use of 'junk science' in defining the problems (S. Milloy, 1995) based on some questionable public health research. The discussion spilled over onto the Internet and the site created by Milloy had, at the time of writing, over four hundred thousand visitors since 1996 and has won a number of awards (www.junkscience.com.) The main issue raised was the danger of believing some opportunistic and dishonest researchers whose main purpose is to acquire financial support or a higher professional status. Some examples include:

- *'one study wonders'* where the statements about the relationships between cause and effect are based on one study without verification by the peers;

- *'science by press conferences'* where the often spurious associations between cause and effect are presented in daily newspapers headlines as facts;

- *'simple causation'* where statements are made about a single cause of a risk or disease which represents a simplified if not a wrong representation of the complex nature of a risk or a disease;

- *'body counts'* where the numbers of people dying from a disease are used to sell the idea of a risk or an exposure to a disease, without accurate indications of the overall population or the time element;

- *'weak associations'* where any association between two variables is accepted without regard to the concept of significance and where the general meaning of 'associations' is confused with 'causation';

- *'modeling'* where any diagram consisting of boxes and arrows is treated as a 'model' and sold as the only respectable way of conceptualising a problem and consequently choosing relevant solutions; such models are usually simplistic, linear and lack any theoretical components; it will be necessary to accept that some events are so complex that no model could provide a satisfactory representation.

The present developments of health promotion and health education practices answer most of the criticism, which may be relevant for some approaches in the past. Raising the subject matter to an academic level is sufficient guarantee that the recommended practices will be based on sound theoretical basis. It will, therefore be necessary to ensure that the practice of health promotion and health education utilizes the recent developments and corrects its past mistakes.

Problems and solutions

Assuming that the methodology is scientifically correct, the next question to be addressed in the future is "what are we studying?" So far most of the studies have been concerned with the distribution and causation of health problems and few studies have addressed the issue of solutions. Once the problem has been defined, health promotion and health education interventions have taken the common-sense approach of telling people what is good for them (cognitive model), in the hope that they will apply the recommendations to their daily life and change their behaviour and actions.

'Variations in health status'

There is a natural variation in health status between individuals and between population groups (defined by geographical location or by social class). This is considered, for political reasons, to be unacceptable and is used as a justification for health actions. There is at present no causal relationship between the recommended actions and these variations and other relevant indicators need to be explored.

The latest developments in information technology (IT) have not as yet been fully exploited by health promotion and health education. The introduction of a settings approach and the concentration on lifestyles has been intended to add **a new dimension to life,** where health is treated as a basic human right and a valuable resource. New developments in IT have introduced a new set of opportunities: they have opened up 'cyberspace' to communications and transfer of information in the form of computer networks, on a global as well as local level. The outcome has been **life in a new dimension** to which people must adjust and the sciences must adapt.

This new dimension has been described differently according to the preferences of the describer. In its widest sense, **cyberspace** is visualized as a dream world where everything is done effectively by computer. One of the supposed advantages of a computer-generated solution is its apparent objectivity and 'best fit' in a well defined situation, since computers can explore all the possible available solutions and chose one that is best for the problem and the situation being tackled. This includes 'virtual reality', which should make life better and avoid unnecessary exposure to the dangers in 'real' reality through simulations. Another way of describing this new dimension is in terms of an **information superhighway** where everybody can communicate with everybody else instantly and continuously by transmitting text, sound and pictures, both moving and still. The most important feature of new information technology is convergence, where the technology of media, information and communication come together to form new opportunities (Baldwin, McVoy and Steinfield, 1996)

The most direct impact of this new dimension is currently made by the **Internet.** This is the world-wide network of linked computers, which is estimated to be used by more than 30 million people. Through the development of the world wide web, it has a wide range of uses, which are constantly growing, and cover practically everything from exchanging scientific information or selling products to exchanging love letters. The presence of health promotion and health education on the Internet is more recent and there is no agreement as to how it should be developed or how it could be used.

Taking health promotion and health education into the 21st century implies developing its theoretical base, concentrating on accountability and exploiting every possible means of communication, including all networks. This is the most recent challenge and its potential needs to be further explored before making a decision whether and how this could be done.

The first issue to be raised is who can have access to the Internet. If one takes into account the global population, then it becomes obvious that only a small proportion has the potential to exploit this new development due to the necessary preconditions (see diagram).

Once access is achieved, the next question is concerned with using the information available. This will be defined by two factors: the position of the receiver to make decisions based on information, and the quality of information necessary for making decisions.

At present, there are many types of Internet presence: commercial enterprises, entertainment, newspapers, special interest groups, hobbyists, pornography purveyors, clubs, children's games and so on. For our purposes, important categories of users are academics and managers, people with a general interest and technical enthusiasts. Academics and researchers use Internet to publicise their area of interest and provide information about their research work. Managers use the Internet to communicate with other managers in the same field, find out what the competition is up to, and promote a high profile for themselves or their company. Technical enthusiasts are individuals obsessed by technology and the Internet provides them with all kind of opportunities to exchange ideas or invade others' private computer space.

Challenge for HP/HE

Any source of information about an activity is important and should be utilized to its full potential. This involves exploring the various ways of how to do it, test it and decide which approaches have been useful, and which represent a waste of time and money. This principle also applies to health promotion and health education use of Internet.

The first question is *"What can we expect from the Internet?"*, and the answer is, that there are a number of advantages which could be gained by using the Internet for the purpose of health promotion and health education. These will depend on the kind of activity and the stage of development. Some of these advantages are:

- in the first stage of the planning process it is useful to have information about the work of others in the chosen field; this should indicate the priority given to a problem, the aspects of the problem which are being addressed and the extent of the inquiry being carried out;

- during the planning process proper, it would be useful to gain information about the methods and the instruments used by others doing similar research; here the problem is that this is rarely available from researchers during the process of their research; for this, one has to wait for the conclusion of a research project, when the report will probably include the methodology and the instruments, although maybe not in sufficient detail to be useful to others; nevertheless, methodologies are also discussed on the Internet;

- when planning an intervention, it is possible to make use of the experience of others in the decision about which methods promise to produce positive outcomes; this kind of information will be only available if the interventions of others have been properly evaluated; unfortunately, many interventions are not properly evaluated, or even if they are, often do not provide the answer to why they were successful but only whether they were judged successful or not;

- the possible spin-off from information about other people's research and interventions may influence the priority given to a problem; a high profile problem is more likely to attract attention and funds (e.g. AIDS) than a more mundane problem (e.g. TB), which may be more important from the point of view of incidence;

- the world-wide information about the standards of research and interventions may provide a bench-mark for others, thus ensuring the quality as well as the quantity of efforts invested in solving health problems through health promotion and health education.

These are a few of the points that should draw the attention of the practitioners in this field to the advantages of using the available information on the Internet to aid their work. The suggestions should serve to motivate people active in this field to get linked to the Internet and make use of the World Wide Web as a part of the planning and execution of their activities.

The other question to be asked is *"What do users of the Internet expect from us?"*, and the answer is, that for the Internet and its available services to be useful in the field of health promotion and health education, practitioners in this field will have to change their approaches and improve the quality of their work. These are some of the changes and improvements, which could help others in using the Internet for their work:

- to be able to use the available information it will be necessary to understand and interpret this information, as well as to be sufficiently critical to assess whether it is acceptable and meets accepted scientific standards; this will require appropriate training of practitioners in the subjects of research and intervention methodologies; a shared common language in this field will be the result of training programmes, standardised in terms of quantity and quality, expressed in the appropriate curricula;

- for others to use it, the information should be made freely available and of a quality useful to others; this will require a greater rigour in the planning and evaluation of health promotion and health education programmes, supported by tested methods and evaluated outcomes;

- the stake-holders have an important role to play in raising the standards of health promotion and health education practices, by setting the specifications for the quality and outcomes of programmes for which they provide finances and support.

These are some of the issues, which represent the challenge to health promotion and health education in the future global communication society. Internet can make information available world-wide, but the quality and usefulness of such information as is available will depend on the quality of the work of individual practitioners and researchers in the field.

Implications for HP/HE

Policy implications

WHO EURO has provided the impetus for the change of emphasis from a problem oriented (medical) approach to a setting (organizational) approach. The next steps to be taken, in order to adjust health promotion policy to this new situation can, therefore, be summarised as follows:

- It will be necessary to take steps to **adjust the existing conceptual framework** of health promotion to include the organizational, as well as the medical model; this will require the inclusion of the existing organizational theories and management methods into health promotion interventions, as well as the development of new ones relevant to looking at health problems within their settings.

- It will also be necessary to **clarify the difference** between the existing practice of health promotion in a setting and the new concept of a 'health promoting setting'. This will need the definition of standards required for the achievement of the status of a health promoting setting and the agreement on specifications concerning the activities;

- Any policy statement should include the **distinction between the role definition** of the health promotion specialist and the role definition of other agents who are expected to be active within the framework of a multisectoral approach for the improvement of health in a population. This implies revising the existing curricula for the purpose of complementing the competence of health promotion specialists in dealing with other professions and settings, as well as the integration of health promotion knowledge and skills into the training programmes of other professions within their own setting.

- The emphasis given to health promotion reflects the scarcity of **empirical studies** related to the application of various concepts and approaches included in practical health promotion. It is still often the case that innovations are promoted due to their ideological or commonsense value without any empirical evidence of their consequences. The clarification of the role of health promotion, as compared to health education, is of vital importance and should be reflected in intervention studies which monitor and evaluate both health promotion and health education aspects.

Strategy Implications

It is not easy to redefine activities (such as health education and health promotion) that were not well defined to start with, and that have achieved recognition only in health promotion circles, whereas other professions often consider them to be either a part of their work (anyway) or basic common sense (using the cognitive model).

In summary, however, the strategy of new health promotion in spite of existing difficulties, should develop two approaches:

- Use the ensuing upheaval arising from the switch of emphasis and **raise the standard of expectations** related to health promotion in general. This can be achieved by means of intervention studies, which are a precondition for the acquisition of a recognised 'health promoting setting' status. They should provide a theoretical basis, which has so far been limited as far as the practice of health promotion is concerned. This has been the main cause of doubt about health promotion's credentials as far as the other more 'respectable' professions were concerned. Once this theoretical base has been provided, it will be relatively easy to include the subject matter into the curricula of other professions who will accept health promotion as a 'normal' part of their activities together with other aspects of their professional practices.

- Use the existing 'pioneering' spirit to recruit as many different settings into the movement, and **set strict standards** for the achievement of recognition of the desired status of a health promoting setting, thus raising the value of the status and not allowing it to be achieved "on the cheap". This will require a clear distinction between health promotion in a setting and a health promoting setting. This, in fact, represents the qualitative difference between the existing and newly recommended practice.

These procedures should shape a viable strategy for the introduction of new health promotion strategies. In summary, it can be stated that in many instances and for many problems, the new approaches of health promotion are the only available solution.

Chapter 2

THE SETTINGS APPROACH

Introduction
The health promoting setting
Workshops for staff

The introduction of a settings approach within an organizational model of health promotion and health education (HP/HE) provided practitioners with a framework which has been considerably more elaborate than the traditional cause-effect approach. An example of a health promoting setting is presented in the following diagram:

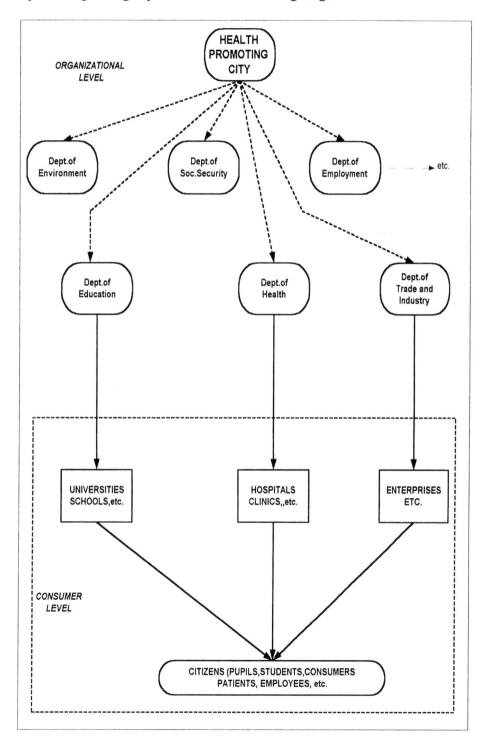

This approach has provided the practitioners with two options:

- To improve the existing planning and execution of HP/HE programmes by taking into consideration the characteristics of a particular setting, its potentials and its requirements; and

- To take the approach to its logical conclusion and transform the setting into a health promoting setting, where the structure and the functions of the setting will reflect the needs of people in terms of their health gain.

Health promotion and health education within a health promoting setting operates on two levels:

- The organizational level

- The consumer level.

The main principle in defining a health promoting setting requires a systems approach within which a health promoting setting is composed of health promoting parts.

This section deals with the issue of taking the approach to its logical conclusion and presents the means of effecting this kind of transformation in creating a health promoting setting and enabling people in such a setting to look after their own health. This can only be achieved through a specific educational programme for the various members of staff within a setting.

The switch to a settings approach is of a recent origin and the newly created health promoting settings are few in number and have not been operating long, so there has hardly been enough time to evaluate this development. It is still the case that most health promotion and health education is only partially and opportunistically integrated into various settings.

The transition of a setting into a health promoting setting includes organizational restructuring relevant to undertaking the following commitments:

- creating a healthy environment,

- integrating HP/HE into the process,

- outreach into community in the form of networks and alliances.

This is usually carried out in three phases: *groundwork, implementation on the organizational level,* and *implementation on the client level.* Most of the existing health promoting settings have more or less successfully completed the first two stages (Grossmann & Scala, 1993), but it is still necessary to find out how the process can be successfully implemented on the client level before one can pass any conclusive judgement on the movement.

At present, there are European networks of different health promoting settings such as healthy cities, health promoting hospitals and health promoting schools. There are also initiatives in the UK. to explore the possibilities of creating 'health promoting general practices', 'health promoting general dental practices', 'health promoting community care system', 'health promoting voluntary organizations', 'health promoting prison' and others.

Creating a health promoting setting

Each of the three phases can be identified with the stages of transforming a setting into a health promoting setting and can be further subdivided into a number of steps, which are set out below:

PHASE 1: GROUNDWORK

This phase is concerned with work at the top administrative and managerial level of a setting, where the decisions are made about the transformation into a health promoting setting. It can be divided into following stages:

Stage 1.1 Consultations

The top management of a setting will have to be convinced that the planned transformation of their setting into a health promoting setting is necessary, feasible and promising in terms of health benefits for the consumers/clients and financial benefits for the setting. These managers should, therefore, be well informed about commitments and possible outcomes as well as the necessary requirements for such an undertaking. The decision should be made about whether they wish to engage in such a process. In the case of a positive decision, the top management will have to undertake a number of commitments and create a Programme

Team, which has the task of initiating the necessary developments and keeping top management informed.

Stage 1.2 Base Line Studies

Once the senior management has agreed that such a transformation is desirable, it will be necessary to establish which problems are to be faced and solved by such a programme.

For this purpose it will be necessary to collect information, using a case study approach (qualitative analysis) and a survey approach (quantitative and secondary data analysis), of the setting and its health problems. Both of these approaches are a part of the assessment process described in detail in Section 6 of this book.

Stage 1.3 Publicity

Depending on the decision made by the senior management in the setting it will be necessary to publicise the changes among staff.

Stage 1.4 Recruitment Programme

The outcome of this ground work should be the implementation of the transformation programme. This will depend on the facilitators (health consultants) who should enable the appropriate programme to be carried out. The health consultants should meet the following criteria:

- have knowledge about health problems (causes and solutions);
- have knowledge and skills in people and resource management;
- have knowledge and skills in HP/HE methods.

Stage 1.5 Workshops for Health Consultants

The selected health consultants should have an opportunity through workshops to learn more about the specific transformation programme, exchange opinions and produce suggestions for its improvement. They should also have an opportunity to update their knowledge in areas in which they do not feel fully competent.

PHASE 2: IMPLEMENTATION ON THE ORGANIZATIONAL LEVEL

This phase includes the Programme Team's advice to the top management, based on the preparatory work concerning the necessary steps that the management needs to undertake, and the extension to various organizational units within the setting, which have agreed to participate in the programme. This will include the following stages (applicable according to the size of the organization):

Stage 2.1 Explanation of Commitments

The organization's top management will have to be briefed about the character of the programme for transforming the setting into a health promoting setting and be invited to prepare consultations with their line managers and employees.

Stage 2.2 Role Distribution

The members of the setting and the management need to decide on a number of issues for the implementation of the transformation programme including the following:

- establishment of needs for the employees for each of the units in the setting; and the selection of topics according to these needs;
- creation of Health Circles and role distribution among its members;
- development of a time table for each specific plan of action;
- deciding on the method of assessment (quality assessment) and the development of a feed-back mechanism for dealing with possible problems.

Stage 2.3 Workshop for Staff

The implementation of a HP/HE programme for the creation of a health promoting setting will require a certain expertise, best obtained by attending a workshop. In the case of smaller organizations, a workshop could be organized for the members of each one of them at the same place, preferably in an educational institution, that is already engaged in providing such training. Once the organizational preconditions have been met the programme can be implemented.

PHASE 3: IMPLEMENTATION ON THE CONSUMER LEVEL

In this phase, the actual HP/HE work takes place. It can take a number of forms and the stages can run consecutively or simultaneously according to the needs and available resources.

Stage 3.1 Plan of Action

According to the established needs of the setting and each of its units, the plan of action will include the following:

- selection of topics and preparation of background material;
- selection of methods according to the topic;
- monitoring and assessment.

Stage 3.2 Implementation

The implementation of the plan of action will include the following:

- the time table, membership, place and the programme of action;
- expert support and relevant material;
- mechanisms for assessment.

The accountability should be ensured by carrying out assessment as a part of the planning process, implementing Total Quality Management as a method of monitoring the process, and evaluation and audit as a part of the measurement of outcome. Where a Quality Management System (QMS) exists it will be possible to add health indicators and specifications. In case where there is no QMS it will be necessary to introduce a specific QMS for HP/HE.

Defining aims and objectives

There is a qualitative difference between health promotion in a setting and a health promoting setting. The 'health promoting setting' is recognised as a special type of setting in terms of its commitments to promoting health in a specific way. The main characteristics of a health promoting setting are a recognised status, an approved and monitored programme, total involvement of the staff, participation in a network of similar settings as well as the creation of alliances with other settings in the community.

The commitment of the management and personnel of a setting should take the form of a policy statement, which should include the following obligations:

- creation of a healthy working and living environment for the members of that setting and the consumers of the products or services of the setting;

- integration of health promotion and health education into the policy, production process and assessment of the settings' activities;

- out-reach into community by means of networks and alliances with other settings and thus contributing to the overall improvement of health of people in that community.

Once the preliminary organizational commitments have been undertaken, people in settings need to define their aims and objectives. The character of the setting will define in greater detail the appropriate aims, objectives, indicators, methods and criteria.

An **aim** describes *what* is intended to be achieved, while an **objective** defines *how* this aim is to be achieved. **Indicators** describe what is considered to be the appropriate way to measure the achievements related to the institution's performance.

Each objective should be followed by a description of the health promotion and health education **methods** that should be used in achieving the set aim, by means of each specific objective. The character of work performed by staff and the services offered to clients should define the specific methods appropriate for the achievement of each aim. The methods available can be differentiated according to the expected outcomes and should include *enabling, mediating and advocating* for the health gain of the staff and clients.

The measurement of the achievements will depend on the validity and reliability of the methods used for each objective. These should not be confused with the validity and reliability of the research instruments (validity refers to whether the instrument actually measures what it is intended to, and reliability refers to the repeatability of results from an instrument by different researchers). *Validity* of HP/HE methods will indicate the possibility or probability of the achievement of a specific aim through the chosen objective and the methods used. *Reliability* of a HP/HE method will indicate the level of success or failure in a general application of chosen methods associated with the objective for the achievement of a specific aim. The interpretation of the results of assessment of the achievement will depend on the *criteria* used for validating the success or failure of the intervention.

For the purpose of evaluation the activities of a health promoting setting can be defined by a set of general and specific aims:

General Aim 1: Creating a Healthy Environment for Staff and Clients

This general aim operates on the settings level and is concerned with the character of the setting, the working environment it provides for staff and clients as well as the internal and external relationships among the staff, among the clients and between staff and clients.

Specific Aim 1.1: Creating healthy working conditions

Objective 1.1.1: Securing a healthy working environment
    Indicator.1.1.1.1: Level of safety at the work place
        Method (enabling, mediating, advocating):
        Evaluation (criteria):

Objective 1.1.2: Ensuring satisfactory working arrangements
    Indicator 1.1.2.1: Level of complaints by staff and management
        Method (enabling, mediating, advocating):
        Evaluation (criteria):

Objective 1.1.3: Ensuring job satisfaction of staff
    Indicator 1.1.3.1: Level of motivation and turnover of staff
        Method (enabling. mediating, advocating):
        Evaluation (criteria):

Objective 1.1.4: Meeting the needs of the clients
    Indicator 1.1.4.1: Level of need satisfaction of clients
        Method (enabling, mediating, advocating):
        Evaluation (criteria):

Specific Aim 1.2: Proper accommodation for staff and clients

Objective 1.2.1: Ensuring proper accommodation for staff
    Indicator 1.2.1.1: Level of staff satisfaction
        Method (enabling, mediating, advocating):
        Evaluation (Criteria):

Objective 1.2.2: Ensuring proper accommodation for clients
    Indicator 1.2.2.1: Level of complaints by clients
        Method (enabling, mediating, advocating):
        Evaluation (Criteria):

Objective 1.2.3: Ensuring appropriate commuting facilities
    Indicator 1.2.3.1: Level of complaints about commuting
        Method (enabling, mediating, advocating):
        Evaluation (Criteria):

Objective 1.2.4: Ensuring alternative accommodation
    Indicator 1.2.4.1: Utilisation of alternative accommodation
        Method (enabling, mediating, advocating):
        Evaluation (Criteria):

Specific Aim 1.3: Availability of healthy nutrition for staff and clients

Objective 1.3.1: Assessment of existing nutritional values
    Indicator 1.3.1.1: Meeting standards for healthy nutrition
        Method (enabling, mediating, advocating):
        Evaluation (Criteria):

Objective 1.3.2: Provision of a healthy diet
    Indicator 1.3.2.1: Selection of food on offer
        Method (enabling, mediating, advocating):
        Evaluation (Criteria):

Objective 1.3.3: Improvements in the catering system
    Indicator 1.3.3.1: level of competence of catering staff
        Method (enabling, mediating, advocating):
        Evaluation (Criteria):

Specific Aim 1.4: Prevention and treatment

Objective 1.4.1: Prevention of health threats for staff
    Indicator 1.4.1.1: Changes in health behaviour of staff
        Method (enabling, mediating, advocating):
        Evaluation (Criteria):

Objective 1.4.2: Prevention of health threats for clients
    Indicator 1.4.2.1: Changes in health behaviour of clients
        Method (enabling, mediating, advocating):
        Evaluation (criteria):

Objective 1.4.3: Utilisation of preventive services by staff
    Indicator 1.4.3.1: Level of utilisation
        Method (enabling, mediating, advocating):
        Evaluation (Criteria):

Objective 1.4.4: Utilisation of preventive services by clients
    Indicator 1.4.4.1: Level of utilization
        Method (enabling, mediating, advocating):
        Evaluation (Criteria):

Objective 1.4.5: Improvement of services (treatment, teaching, production, etc.)
    Indicator 1.4.5.1: Level of negative outcomes (complaints)
        Method (enabling, mediating, advocating):
        Evaluation (Criteria):

Specific Aim 1.5: Care and relationships

Objective 1.5.1: Improvement of relations between staff
    Indicator 1.5.1.1: Level of conflicts & discriminations
        Method (enabling, mediating, advocating):
        Evaluation (Criteria):

Objective 1.5.2: Improvement in staff - client relations
    Indicator 1.5.2.1: Level of conflict & complaints
        Method (enabling, mediating, advocating):
        Evaluation (Criteria):

Objective 1.5.3: Improvements of relations between clients
    Indicator 1.5.3.1: Level of conflicts
        Method (enabling, mediating, advocating):
        Evaluation (Criteria):

Objective 1.5.4: Improvement in client satisfaction
    Indicator 1.5.4.1 Level of satisfaction of client needs
        Method (enabling, mediating, advocating):
        Evaluation (Criteria):

General Aim 2: Integrating Health Promotion into the Daily Activities in the Setting

This aim operates on the staff-client level, and takes into account the fact that the structure of most settings is composed of a number of units which can be called departments, workplace, production units, subjects, clinics, outlets etc. Each of these units has a separate management structure, specific aims and different people working in it. The integration of health promotion into the daily activities of a setting will, therefore, have to be carried out for each of these units separately.

Specific Aim 2.1: Consideration and satisfaction of the health needs of the staff

Objective 2.1.1: Ensure that the staff avoids risk-creating behaviour
    Indicator 2.1.1.1: Level of smoking, obesity, and other risk-creating behaviours
        Method: (enabling, mediating, and advocating)
        Evaluation (criteria):

Objective 2.1.2: Ensure that staff utilizes preventive services
    Indicator 2.1.2.1: Level of utilization of health services (check-ups, cervical screening, etc.,
        Method (enabling, mediating, advocating):
        Evaluation (criteria):

Objective 2.1.3: Ensure that the staff's working conditions are compliant with reduction of risk at work
 Indicator 2.1.3.1: Level of stress, accidents, , etc., measured indirectly and directly
  Method (enabling, mediating, advocating):
  Evaluation (criteria):
Objective 2.1.4: Ensure the general health of the staff
 Indicator 2.1.4.1: Level of utilization and timing of curative health services
  Method (enabling, mediating, advocating):
  Evaluation (criteria):

Specific Aim 2.2: Consideration and satisfaction of the needs of the clients

Objective 2.2.1: Ensuring the health aspects of services and/or goods provided for clients
 Indicator 2.2.1.1: Level of health hazards associated with the client population
  Method (enabling, mediating, advocating):
  Evaluation (criteria):

Objective 2.2.2: Ensuring the client's awareness of health risks and available solutions
 Indicator 2.2.2.1: Level of client competence in avoidance of risk to health
  Method (enabling, mediating, advocating):
  Evaluation (criteria):

Objective 2.2.3: Ensuring the client's competence in dealing with existing health problems and health risks
 Indicator 2.2.3.1: Level of client's competence
  Method (enabling, mediating, advocating):
  Evaluation (criteria);

Specific Aim 2.3: Assessing and meeting the needs of the immediate social environment

Objective 2.3.1: Ensuring the social support from the client's family and relatives
 Indicator 2.3.1.1: Level of support, conjugal roles, family cycle of development
  Method (enabling, mediating, advocating):
  Evaluation (criteria):

Objective 2.3.2: Ensuring the social support from client's colleagues at work
 Indicator 2.3.2.1: Level of support from colleagues at work
  Method (enabling, mediating, advocating):
  Evaluation (criteria):

Objective 2.3.3: Ensuring the social support from client's reference group, friends and neighbours
 Indicator 2.3.3.1: Level of support
  Method (enabling, mediating, advocating):
  Evaluation (criteria):

General Aim 3: Initiating and participating in community developments

This general aim operates on the settings level and is concerned with the settings position and interactions within the community.

Specific Aim 3.1: Initiating and promoting the "health promoting setting" movement in the community

Objective 3.1.1: Popularising the "health promoting" status of the setting in the community
    Indicator 3.1.1.1: Amount and content analysis of the publicity given to the setting in media
        Method (enabling, mediating, advocating):
        Evaluation (criteria):

Objective 3.1.2: Public meetings for representatives of other settings to learn about the concept of "health promoting settings"
    Indicator 3.1.2.1: Attendance rate, comments and commitments of the attending representatives of other settings
        Method (enabling, mediating, advocating):
        Evaluation (criteria):

Objective 3.1.3: Workshops for representatives of other settings interested in becoming a "health promoting setting"
    Indicator 3.1.3.1: Attendance rate, level of satisfaction and learning achievements, level of commitment
        Method (enabling, mediating, advocating):
        Evaluation (criteria)

Specific Aim 3.2: Networking with other similar health promoting settings

Objective 3.2.1: Creating and/or joining a local network of similar settings
    Indicator 3.2.1.1: Extent of the local network
        Method (enabling, mediating, advocating):
        Evaluation (criteria):

Objective 3.2.2: Creating and/or joining the national network of similar health promoting settings
    Indicator 3.2.2.1: Extent of the national network
        Method (enabling, mediating, advocating):
        Evaluation (criteria);

Objective 3.2.3: Creating and/or joining the international network of similar settings
    Indicator 3.2.3.1: Extent of the international network
        Method (enabling, mediating, advocating):
        Evaluation (criteria):

Specific Aim 3.3: Creating healthy alliances with other health promoting settings on a local, national and international level

Objective 3.3.1: Establishing mechanisms for cooperation with other health promoting settings on a local level (e.g. hospitals, schools, services, enterprises, prisons, etc.)
    Indicator 3.3.1.1: Extent of the cooperation with other settings
        Method (enabling, mediating, advocating):
        Evaluation (criteria):
Objective 3.3.2: Establishing mechanisms for cooperation with other health promoting settings on a national level
    Indicator 3.3.2.1: Extent of cooperation with other settings
        Method (enabling, mediating, advocating):
        Evaluation (criteria):

Objective 3.3.3: Establishing mechanisms for cooperation with other health promoting settings on an international level
    Indicator 3.3.3.1: Extent of cooperation with other settings
        Method (enabling, mediating, advocating):
        Evaluation (criteria):

The detailed description of the three commitments of a health promoting setting, expressed in the form of general aims and supported by specific aims, objectives, indicators and criteria, provides the members of a setting with the opportunity to understand the true meaning of the commitment and the requirements of the expected activities involved in accepting the status of a health promoting setting.

Creating a health promoting setting through self-care and self-determination, involves, in the first phase, the popularisation of the movement concerned with declaring certain settings as 'health promoting', and the actions of settings in achieving such improvements. The second phase includes the raising of competence of staff in a setting and/or representatives in four major areas: **initiating, organizing, managing** and **evaluating** the setting's activities.

This example of how to organize a workshop offers a blueprint aimed at raising the competence of staff in a setting. It can be organized by a training institution or, where appropriate, within the setting itself.

The participants of the workshop should be the management and professional staff of settings who have shown an interest in participating in this movement. They would be expected, after attending the Workshop and learning about the requirements for this involvement, to take on the commitment to participate in the movement.

This movement is based on a similar concept of 'health promoting health care system', developed in some European countries, and already spreading, with a number of settings declaring themselves as 'health promoting settings'.

The background qualifications of the participants will be different, ranging from highly educated professionals to management experts and administrative staff.

The teaching programme of the workshop is divided into four modules dealing with the following topics: initiating, organizing, managing and assessing a setting programme.

Workshop Module 1: Initiating A Programme

The **aims** of this module are to enable the participants to become familiar with and competent in 'selling' the idea of declaring their setting as a 'Health Promoting Setting' to the people living in that community, by emphasising the advantages and presenting the realistic contributions expected from each community member and setting staff.

At the end of the initiation period the setting should have established a working team, examined the existing problem and selected the priorities in preparation for the development of the organization programme. The stages of the initiating process include:

The 'Acceptance' Process

Initiating a setting's activity requires the support of the setting's staff, expressed in their active commitment to certain activities. To achieve the general acceptance of the idea of declaring a setting 'health promoting', the first step should be the discussion of the idea and its implications with individual staff members of the setting. This should create awareness of the possibilities as well as responsibilities associated with such a commitment. The individuals should be chosen for their influence, possible opposition, control of resources, etc. At the end of this process, the idea should be known in the setting and the staff should have had the opportunity to sound out the 'significant others' whose opinions they value and respect.

The part of the Workshop Module 1 covering this stage in the process should enable the participants to acquire skills in 'directive interviewing', i.e. individual conversations with the aim of acquainting a partner with the idea and sounding out their opinions and possible objections.

The content should include information about raising issues, listening to opinions, providing arguments, answering questions, as well as about the way of conducting an interview (introduction, questions and answers, conclusion).

The method of acquiring this knowledge, as well as skills, related to interviewing should include simple explanation of the major points, supported by numerous illustrations and followed by practice in the form of role play.

The assessment should include the expression of confidence by the participants, the opinions of their partners and the external observers, as well as the assessment of the supervisor.

Mass Meeting

Following the general preparation, the initiating process should include the organization of a mass meeting of the setting staff. This can be a special meeting or a part of an existing mass meeting. The organization includes the following stages:

- the advertising of the meeting, including the title, the time, the place, the agenda and the speakers;

- the agenda should include the clarification of the concept, the outline of advantages and possible disadvantages and the role distribution of potential participants;

- the 'questions and answers' period should be allowed sufficient time for clarification of any issues and constructive treatment of any objections;

- the outcome of the meeting should be the acceptance by people within the setting as a whole to undertake the commitment and enter into the exploratory process of finding out in reality what this commitment implies;

- the follow-up should sound out individuals according to the role definition presented as part of the agenda, and organize a meeting with the members who agreed to participate actively in attempts to improve the 'life' of the setting, which could also include health issues.

The part of the Workshop Module 1 covering the organization of a mass meeting should enable participants to acquire skills in planning, advertising, organizing, leading and participating in such meetings. The contents should include information about attracting attention and using mass media; the considerations to be taken into account when planning a meeting, including place, size of the auditorium, seating arrangements, acoustics, lighting, chairing and running a meeting, presentation of speeches, leading a discussion, answering questions, dealing with troublemakers, and getting a commitment or opinion by sounding out the participants. The method of acquiring this knowledge and skills should include some general advice, a task and role-play. The assessment should include the subjective feelings of the participants and subsequent evaluation of the meetings organized by the participants.

Forming a Working Team

The individuals concerned with the issue and willing actively to support the movement who come to the smaller meeting following the mass meeting, should deal with the following topics:

- forming 'working teams' in various parts of the setting from among all the people interested;

- distributing the tasks among the members in relation to the organizational programme;

- taking on the task of studying and defining the problems in the setting.

The part of Workshop Module 1 dealing with forming working teams should enable the participants individually to approach different members at the mass meeting, recruit them for a working team and distribute tasks among them. The contents should include the understanding of the rationale for building such a team, familiarity with the general problems of the setting, the skills in collecting and storing information, ability to assess the potential contributions of each member, gaining their commitment and setting the task of objectively establishing the problems in the setting. The method should include some simple explanations about team leadership; practical skills in collecting and storing data, data analysis, and presenting the findings in an interesting and relevant way; these skills should be acquired during the work on tasks and practical examples. The assessment should be based on the preparations for the next mass meeting and reaction of the staff to the presentations; it should also be based on the choice of priorities and the level of commitment of the staff.

Second Mass Meeting

Once the work of the teams has been completed, they should call another mass meeting to discuss the findings and inform all the setting staff about the progress made towards organizing certain activities. The outcome of this meeting should be a general agreement of the setting about the priority of problems according to their seriousness and feasibility.

The part of Workshop Module 1, dealing with organizing the second mass meeting, should enable the participants to learn from the experiences gained during the organization of the first mass meeting and avoid most of the mistakes made. The contents should include ways of critically analysing the outcomes and possible improvements. The method should include the simulation process in the form of tasks, where the participants get information about an imaginary meeting and carry out the exercise of improving on it. The assessment should be based on the outcome of the exercises as well as on the level of confidence expressed by the participants. A long-term assessment should include the evaluation of the second mass meeting.

These preparations should produce a programme of future activities and Workshop Module 2 deals with its planning and organization.

Workshop Module 2: Programme Planning and Organization

Once the general idea of commitment has been understood and the staff have expressed their readiness to participate in this 'movement', the **aims** of this workshop module are to enable the participants to become competent and confident in drafting a programme for action, testing it with the general staff of the setting and producing a final organizational and operational programme for action.

The first step in planning and organizing a programme for action should be to make a diagnosis by examining the causes and prescribing relevant solutions. The 'medical' diagnosis should be available from the medical profession and it should include medical 'causes and solutions'. For a HP/HE intervention it is necessary to carry out a differential diagnosis with the emphasis on 'health promotional/educational solutions'.

One should take into consideration the fact that the activities of a 'Health Promoting Setting' should include the problems of the staff working in the setting, the problems of the clients using the setting and the community within which the setting is located. The solutions to the problems in each of these areas should be adjusted to the needs and possibilities of each one. The success of such a simultaneous set of activities in these interacting areas should require a mechanism for co-ordination, evaluation and feedback. The main steps to be discussed in the workshop can be envisaged as follows:

Commitment

The implementation of the chosen solution should require the agreement and commitment of the institution, the clients and the community concerning certain required actions. This commitment can include resources, working time, expertise, services, etc. The nature and the character of the solutions prescribed should define it.

Tasks

Once the general commitment within the setting has been gained, the next step should be to specify the solutions in terms of activities. These activities should then be distributed in the form of task distributions, for settings, and role definition, for individual members of each setting.

Action

Getting the whole programme under way will require actions on the part of the participants in the setting, following the task distributions and role definitions. These actions will have to be synchronised to achieve maximum effectiveness.

Synchronisation of activities will require a mechanism for coordination as well as close cooperation of all the actors involved.

The task of such a mechanism for co-ordination of a programme will depend on the management skills of the teams, and this is the aim of Workshop Module 3.

Workshop Module 3: Management of the Programme

The **aims** of this module are to enable the participants to acquire knowledge about issues involved in management of a programme as well as skills in carrying it out.

The main objective of management is to *co-ordinate* the various planned activities involving members of the setting and their patients. This co-ordination is vital for *simultaneous actions* to take place.

Some of the solutions will depend for their success on the *synchronicity* of actions, such as for example in changing norms, values and opinions of the members of the setting and the patients.

The management of the programme should also include synchronising commitments within the setting as a whole and among its different parts, their acceptance of specific tasks and roles, as well as the adjustments of their actions with the aim of supporting and reinforcing each other. Success should be evaluated. This is dealt with in Workshop Module 4.

Workshop Module 4: Evaluation and Feedback

The **aims** of this Workshop Module are to provide the participants with an understanding of the need for and the skills necessary for ensuring the accountability of people engaged in a program, which includes assessment, quality management, and evaluation of an intervention programme, as well as making use of the feedback mechanism for the adjustments and corrections of the programme. It should clarify the distinction between the traditional evaluation process and the new demand for accountability of the agents (see Chapter 6 of this book).

Assessment should be included in the planning stages of an intervention. The intervention process requires a 'quality management mechanism' (or the use of the existing QMS). The outcome should be evaluated and possibly also audited. To achieve a successful evaluation, the following preconditions should be met:

- aims and objectives should be defined in a measurable way; measurement requires a set of indicators, defined by criteria for assessment and translated into instruments to carry out the measurements; quality assessment requires a set of specifications for the expected outcomes, agreed upon by the purchasers, providers and consumers;
- the programme should be divided into steps or phases, and each one should require a specific evaluation of the achievement of each sub-aim or sub-objective;

- the programme should include a mechanism for utilising feedback information and adjusting the programme accordingly;
- in terms of a 'community' type action in a setting, the phases involved are:

i. *Commitment:* It will be necessary critically to assess the commitments undertaken within the setting as a whole as well as by the individual members; these should be synchronised and should be supportive as well as specific; they should also be relevant to the aims of the programme; any problems noted at this stage should be fed back into the system and corrected before the next phase is undertaken;

ii. *Tasks and roles:* It is important to distinguish between the general and specific aspects of commitments; the specific commitments will make task distributions and the role definitions possible; any problems due to the mismatch between the institutional tasks and individual role performance should be fed back into the system and adjustments should be made;

iii. *Actions:* Evaluation should link the commitments undertaken with the distribution of tasks and roles and the actions carried out; it should also link the actions monitored with the actual achievements in terms of programme aims; since a number of actions and activities will be carried out within the framework of the programme aims, each one should be assessed separately; the feedback mechanism should enable corrections and adjustments over time, since action in a setting represents an ongoing programme and continuous activity as part of changing the life style in the setting.

Chapter 3

DEFINITION OF PROBLEMS
AND
CHOICE OF SOLUTIONS

Introduction
Definition of Problems
Choice of Solutions

INTRODUCTION

Health promotion and health education interventions depend on the definition of the problems and the choice of appropriate solutions. In the past, the definition of health problems has been mainly concerned with medical aspects, while the health promotional and health educational aspects have largely been neglected or taken for granted. The consequence has been that the choice of HP/HE solutions has had no direct link to the definition of the problems, since this definition being in medical terms, did not provide any insight into the kind of health promotion and health education intervention necessary for achieving the best results. By default, the preferred health promotional and health educational solutions have been based on a common sense approach, usually applying a cognitive model of the transmission of information, in the hope that the recipient will make an educated decision to take action about the health threat or disease in question.

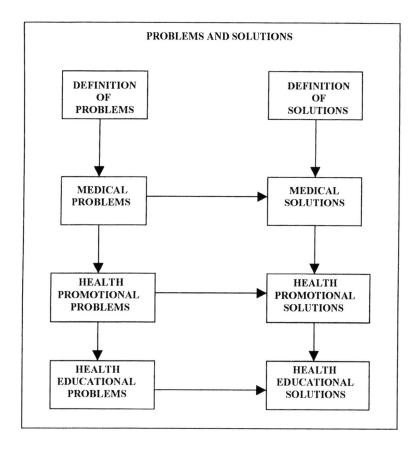

This section draws the distinction between the medical and the health promotional and health educational aspects of problems and solutions. It deals with the specific need for defining the problem and choosing solutions from the point of view of the knowledge and skills necessary for making a differential diagnosis of the problems within a setting, and the choice of appropriate solutions of a HP/HE nature. The differential diagnosis is based on the information about the setting (assessment) and examines the health problems experienced by the people in the setting. The choice of solutions includes interventions by people occupying roles within a setting. Solutions are based on the principles of enabling, mediating and advocating, for the health gain of the consumer. These interventions should be evaluated for the purpose of finding out the level of health gain and possible negative side effects from the intervention.

DEFINITION OF PROBLEMS

Recent advances in medical knowledge and medical technology have extended the definition of health, beyond medical factors, to include also the environmental and personal factors associated with the spread of disease. At the same time, advances in the understanding of social processes and the psychology of individuals have been reflected in the new definition of the problems facing health promotion and health education. For these reasons, those working in health promotion and health education have to consider all these factors when defining the problem that they are aiming to solve, including the following:

- the **medical** aspect of the definition of the problem includes two approaches, the etiological and the epidemiological; the etiological approach looks at the medical, social/environmental and personal factors; the epidemiological approach looks at risk factors and human behaviour;

- the **health promotional** aspect includes the environmental approach and the analysis of the individual adjustment to it; the environmental approach looks at physical, social and organizational factors; the individual adjustment looks at physical and social factors as well as the relationship to available services;

- the **health educational** aspect of the definition of the problem includes approaches based on understanding knowledge, attitudes and skills; the knowledge is concerned with health threats, services and supportive systems; the attitudes to problems and to solutions are examined; the skills to be examined include coping, communication and behaviour modification skills.

Medical Aspects

The medical definition of a health problem will be mainly concerned with the establishment of the causation, which will define the choice of the medical solution. The cause(s) can be discovered by laboratory research (etiology), or if that is not successful, then the probability of causation can be established by the study of the distribution of a problem in a population (epidemiology) and examining the characteristics of the affected population, contributing to the presence of a health problem. In the former case, a mechanism will be discovered which causes the presence of a disease (for example, a bacterium associated with a disease), whereas in the latter case, where an agent cannot be found, a certain population characteristic may indicate the possible association between a characteristic such as a behaviour and a disease (for example smoking and cancer).

Given that the cause of a disease is known, a medical practitioner will be faced with establishing the presence of the disease in a patient, depending on the presented symptoms or complaints. The medical practitioner will have to carry out a differential diagnosis, by excluding irrelevant information and deciding which of the many possible diseases best fits the presented pattern of symptoms and complaints. Following the diagnosis, a treatment will be prescribed.

The contribution made by an appropriate medical diagnosis is of great importance for the approach and the contents of a health promotion and health education intervention. The approach will be influenced by the way the medical definition has been carried out. If the cause is known and is directly linked to the disease, the approach can be directed at individuals who are at higher than average risk of being exposed to the agent that causes the disease, with the aim of preventing or helping in the management and treatment of the disease. If the cause is only presumed, by virtue of an association between certain population characteristics and the presence of the disease, the approach will in general be directed towards the population, since it is not possible to translate a population probability to an individual case. The contents of health promotion and health education will reflect the existing medical knowledge about the causation, prevention and management of a disease.

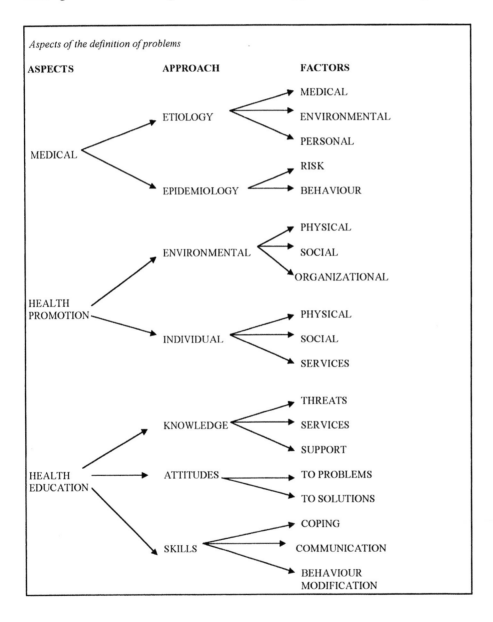

Aspects of the definition of problems

ASPECTS	APPROACH	FACTORS
MEDICAL	ETIOLOGY	MEDICAL / ENVIRONMENTAL / PERSONAL
	EPIDEMIOLOGY	RISK / BEHAVIOUR
HEALTH PROMOTION	ENVIRONMENTAL	PHYSICAL / SOCIAL / ORGANIZATIONAL
	INDIVIDUAL	PHYSICAL / SOCIAL / SERVICES
HEALTH EDUCATION	KNOWLEDGE	THREATS / SERVICES / SUPPORT
	ATTITUDES	TO PROBLEMS / TO SOLUTIONS
	SKILLS	COPING / COMMUNICATION / BEHAVIOUR MODIFICATION

Thus, health promotion and health education will benefit from medical research concerned with the definition of the problem, and in addition will be able to contribute to the effectiveness of diagnosis by sensitizing the patient to the important signals or signs the body provides as an indication of a disease.

Etiology

The history of medicine is characterized by changes in the assumptions concerning the causation and the character of disease and the means of their cure. The beliefs of yesterday are obsolete today; and today's beliefs will almost certainly be obsolete tomorrow. The progression of our understanding of disease, as well as its prevention and management, follows the general pattern of scientific development with all its potentials, doubts, uncertainties and mistakes. It is important to bear this in mind when talking about the way a health threat, or a disease, can be prevented and/or treated.

It is important to understand this complex picture in considering the medical definition of health problems (McKeown,1977). It is often assumed that definitions are clear-cut and can be derived from examining the medical literature. In doing this, however, one soon discovers the uncertainty and controversies, even within the medical profession, about such definitions. Defining a problem in medical terms is vital for health promotion and education purposes, provided the processes by which the medical profession arrived at their definitions are understood. Since a doctor cannot be absolutely certain in most cases about the accuracy of the diagnosis, as well as the effectiveness of the treatment, he or she must learn to cope with uncertainty. The problem of uncertainty can be reduced by continuous contact between the doctor and the patient, which will enable the doctor to react to the feedback during the treatment and adjust it accordingly.

Taking these reservations into account, the etiology or causation of a health problem can be analysed according to current knowledge, which includes the causal agent, the means of acquisition and/or transmission, the incubation period, the symptoms, the process and the expected outcome. These aspects make up a life-style system. They can be differentiated according to the main characteristics of the following factors relevant for health promotion and health education:

1. Medical Factors: From a whole range of medical factors that are relevant to the diagnosis, management and treatment of a disease, it is possible to highlight those directly relevant to a health education or promotion intervention:

- *causal factors* are generally considered to be those which deal with the mode of acquisition and/or transmission of the disease in terms of specific agents or processes which are currently associated with that particular disease;
- *risk factors* are generally considered to be those which have been found to contribute to the increased probability of acquiring or transmitting a disease.

2. Social/environmental factors: These are the external factors that have been found to be associated with the acquisition or transmission of certain diseases, originating in:

- *the physical environment,* related to air, water, food, climate, pests, transport, communication, etc.;

- *the social environment*, determining the social position of the target population, including their income and occupation, culture and religion, their value and belief systems, norms and role performance, available services, access to professional help, etc.

3. Personal factors: Within a given physical and social environment, people, individually or in groups, may act, or react, differently to health threats, or the availability of existing resources. These individuals and groups will have specific characteristics, which are associated with their genetic makeup, their exposure to certain risk factors, their competence in dealing with a health problem and their preference for the choices available. The personality and the competence of individuals will be reflected in:

- *life style*, which has been found to be associated with the probability of acquiring and transmitting certain diseases;
- *habits and routines*, which represent learned reactions to certain stimuli, and can be associated with the incidence of certain diseases;
- *actions*, which may or may not take place, and which can be associated with certain diseases.

Epidemiology

Epidemiology, or the study of the distribution of a disease in a population, has made some major contributions to the understanding of the causation of diseases. It has raised a number of other important issues associated with planning the provision of health care, the protection of human rights associated with inequalities in health and the treatment of disease, and the influence of the environment (physical and social) on the health of a population.

The distribution of a disease in a population is associated with the distribution of certain medical, social/environmental and personal factors within that population. It is useful to define as a system the community/group at risk or the 'target' population. The distribution of risk factors is of particular interest in health education and promotion.

1. Risk factors: The distribution of different risk factors, associated with a health threat or a disease, is of importance for the definition of a population at risk in health education and health promotion terms. This can be achieved by studying the characteristics of the overall population and identifying the segment that manifests the presence of certain risk factors. The different levels of risk are associated with the distribution of the following types of risk factors in a population, which are usually interrelated and need not be mutually exclusive:

- *environmental* risk factors such as air or water pollution, can contribute to the spread of a disease;
- *socio-economic* risk factors include housing, income, employment, social class, education and a number of other factors that have been found to be associated with the prevalence of a health threat or disease in a population;
- *behavioural* risk factors, including smoking, diet, leisure, stressful life style, alcohol and drug abuse, certain patterns of sexual activities and other aspects associated with individual attitudes and behaviour related to health and disease.

2. Behaviour: One of the main determinants of risk from a certain health threat or disease is people's behaviour. The distribution of different kinds of behaviour in a population will help in defining the target population for health education and health promotion interventions. The types of behaviour related to the definition of a medical problem are:

- *orientation to health care*, which can differ according to the 'parochial' or 'cosmopolitan' characteristics of the population (Suchman 1965) ;
- *utilisation of health services*, which depends on people's relationship with the health professions and the amount of self confidence and competence they have in dealing with health problems;
- *perception of health threats*, which is associated with the socio-economic and educational characteristics of a population.

These general characteristics of people's behaviour can be subdivided in terms of its relation to the health problems as:

- *health related behaviour* - which includes all types of behaviour directly or indirectly associated with a health threat or a diseases; and
- *health directed behaviour* - which is specifically aimed at improving health or avoiding disease.

Health Promotional Aspects

Health promotion is mainly concerned with the environment in which a person or a population lives, and with the ability of a person to adjust to this environment or to change it as necessary.

Environmental factors

The definition of an existing problem for a health promotion intervention will have to include an examination of certain environmental factors, which will affect the level of people's self-reliance and competence in dealing with a health threat or a disease. These factors include the physical environment, the social environment and organizational structures.

1. Physical environment: There are many characteristics of people's physical environment, which can be a cause of a disease or a contributing factor to its spread and persistence. Some of the more obvious characteristics such as climatic conditions, communication and transportation systems, etc., will require different health promotion interventions:

- some will be aimed at raising people's competence in adjusting to the living conditions;
- others will be concerned with changing these conditions, and reducing the adverse effects on people's health.

2. Social environment: Norms or social expectations reflect the predominant value system in a community, associated with the way people deal with a health threat or disease. These norms can be related to:

- *life style*, which reflects the individual's position in a society, values and beliefs, behaviour and actions, and the ranking order of preferences or issues of importance, which together can be subsumed under the general concept of a life style;

- *risky behaviour*, which refers to specific forms of behaviour or action associated with an increased risk from a health threat or a disease; generally speaking, this risky behaviour will reflect types of social norms and specific norm characteristics (historicity, social support, sanctions etc.);
- *support systems*, which are complementary to the health care system, and originate in the community to provide knowledge, skills and support in the form of self-help groups. An examination of the existing supportive services as well as those, which could be helpful if they existed, will contribute to the definition of the problem in health promotional terms.

3. Organizational structures: The existing organizational and administrative bodies, which will be relevant for a health threat or a disease, will include medical services associated with management and treatment, as well as other supportive systems. These will be relevant for the following:

- *diagnosis* of the problem, which will include the presence of risk factors, which can be medical or behavioural; covers screening services, as well as studies carried out by the public health services;
- *treatment* in health promotional terms, including operating with social policies and norms, and the creation of new services, or the reinforcement of existing services, which will be influenced by the distribution of a risk factor or a disease in a population;
- *utilization* of services, reflecting the types of norms related to dealing with a specific health threat or disease.

Individual adjustment

Individuals and groups will be exposed to different kinds of health threats and diseases within the same social environment. This is highly relevant to defining a problem in health promotional terms, and needs to be incorporated in the aims and objectives of a health promotional intervention. There are various important areas in which individual adjustment must be made.

1. The physical environment: The way in which individuals cope with the environment depends on their awareness of its dangers, as well as their confidence in being able to affect it and improve it. Health promotion has an important role in raising people's competence in dealing with environmental issues either individually or through some other social mechanisms.

2. The social environment: Even where there are social expectations aimed at reducing risk and preventing a disease, individual perception of those expectations or norms may be decisive for the type of behaviour or action within a certain life style that is in operation. This perception may be related to the following aspects of norms:

- *the accurate interpretation* of existing expectations relevant to the situation in which an individual finds himself/herself;
- *existing legitimization*, which includes the professional as well as lay support for behaviour conforming to a norm;
- *existing sanctions*, which are associated with the deviant behaviour related to a norm.

3. Services: Even where certain services exist, they may not be known, accessible or attractive enough to individuals or groups, which could reduce their utilisation. In health promotional terms, is necessary to define any problems related to the utilisation of the following services:

- *preventive services,* which may include screening services, antenatal clinics etc. aimed at preventing certain health threats or diseases;
- *management services,* which can include certain types of hospitals, as well as self-help groups;
- *treatment services,* which may include general practitioners, hospitals, and certain outlets for paramedical services and complementary medicine.

Health Educational Aspects

For years, the attempts to improve people's health by means of education have been the main responsibility of health education. With the introduction of the concept of health promotion, it became necessary to redefine health education within this new framework. Health education is the process of transmission and/or acquisition of knowledge and skills, on an individual or group level, which are necessary for survival and for the improvement of the quality of life. There are many definitions, each emphasizing different aspects of this process. Some definitions include both the individual approach and the community approach, which is the collective effort to attain health.

According to the above definition, the health educational intervention will be limited to dealing with individuals and groups, in contrast to the health promotional intervention, which deals with societal factors. Drawing these demarcation lines between health education and health promotion requires a specific approach to the definition of a problem in health educational terms. In taking this view, the definition of the health educational aspects of a health problem should consider a number of factors, such as those set out below.

Knowledge

Awareness of or knowledge about the existence of a health threat or a disease is considered to be an important, although not absolutely necessary, precondition for prevention, management and treatment on an individual or group basis. Most health education interventions concentrate on improving the methods of transmitting information and knowledge about the causes of diseases, and the means of preventing them. With the expansion of health education in industrial societies, it soon became apparent that even with considerable knowledge, the prevalence of certain diseases has not been reduced. Further studies have found that health-related and health-directed behaviour is a function of a number of factors, of which knowledge is only one. With the present revolution in the field of information technology, the transmission of knowledge/information has developed a new importance. In the past, knowledge and information were aimed at specific individuals, and surveys of individuals were used to evaluate effectiveness in transmitting health education messages. New technology has given whole communities, countries or the global society instantaneous access to knowledge/information. The fact that a whole population can receive an item of information simultaneously suggests that this can be instrumental in changing the value system or norms of that society or community. This gives the transmission of knowledge a new role – it is important, not so much because it increases individual knowledge about the diseases, and the means of prevention and management, but because it affects the value system and norms related to health behaviour and actions in a population.

On an individual level, nevertheless, it is important to examine existing knowledge or awareness about the following:

- *Health threats and diseases:* Although everybody is exposed to all the health threats and diseases that are prevalent in a society, some people are more exposed than others. In this sense, the knowledge about relative probability associated with a health threat or a disease should provide a positive motivation for adjustment and changes.
- *Services:* The knowledge about the existence and the availability of certain services can be an important precondition for their utilization. This includes, not only knowledge about the existence of a service and its character, but also such details as address and telephone number, transport, hours of work, available personnel etc. It will also include the type of services provided, and the expectations that a certain service should meet.
- *Support systems:* The awareness of existing support systems, which can be organised through the health care system (anti-smoking clinic) or by self-help groups (mothers with handicapped children), is an important precondition for their utilization. Awareness about their existence, as well as details about their character and provision of support, will help people to decide about their utilization.

Attitudes

There has been disappointment with the attempts to improve health by means of increasing individuals' levels of knowledge. As a consequence, emphasis has been placed on the way people felt about a health threat and the measures necessary for preventing it. The accent has been put on people's feelings, expressed in their attitudes, which became the main target of health educational interventions.

Today we are aware of the importance of attitudes in the decision making process, but not solely because they represent people's feelings about health actions. They are also important because they represent people's internalization of social expectations (norms), as a part of the more general value system concerning a health issue. This implies that in a society where there are norms (social expectations) which support a positive preventive action, people with positive attitudes towards that action will be labeled as conformists, and will be more likely to undertake such an action. Those with negative attitudes will be labeled deviants, and health education will have the task of changing the deviants into conformists, or to change social expectations (norms). This involves a different approach, compared with the attempts in the past to change people's attitudes on an individual level. Many of such attempts failed, because the changed attitudes were not accompanied by supportive norms, and those people who did change became deviants.

Bearing in mind this new interpretation of the importance of attitudes for health behaviour and actions, people's attitudes or orientation towards certain risk factors or diseases will be important indicators for planning a health education intervention. Attitudes relate to problems and solutions:

- *Attitudes towards problems:* Some problems have acquired a certain image, which is reflected in the attitudes that people have towards them. Some health problems have the image of a killer disease (cancer), carry a social stigma (sexually transmitted diseases), or are associated with particular life styles (coronary heart disease). Attitudes towards different problems may enhance or inhibit people's decisions about changes in life styles or behaviours. This in turn affects their prevention and management.

- *Attitudes towards solutions:* There is a difference between the motivational power of attitudes relating to a problem and a solution. Even if the attitude is positive in terms of action because of the problem's severity and a person's susceptibility to it, a negative attitude towards the solution may act as an inhibiting factor. The cost-benefit assessment of the proposed solution, supported by a positive attitude, may act as a motivational cue to trigger a change in people's life style or behaviour.

Skills

Reducing a health threat, or preventing an illness, may often depend on people's competence, which includes possessing skills required to affect the problem. The definition of these skills and the information about their distribution in a population, are relevant to planning a health education intervention. Among the skills making up people's competence, the following are considered to be important:

- *Coping skills:* The awareness of any health threat or risk from a disease, whether imposed from outside or due to internal factors, represents an upheaval, calling for coping skills. These involve avoiding a certain threat, reducing it, or integrating it positively into a life style.

- *Communication skills:* Individuals and groups must communicate with each other and with the professionals if they are to learn about a health threat or disease or to mobilize support and get help. There are a number of aspects of skills involved in a process of communication, which may include linguistic abilities and coping with social barriers. Defining the problem in this area is of importance for planning any health education intervention.

- *Behaviour modification skills:* Even where there are appropriate levels of knowledge and positive attitudes to the problem and its solution, there are additional skills, needed to enable individuals to modify their life style or behaviour, which can be learned and practised. Information about the lack of those skills should be taken into account when planning a health education intervention.

Introduction

Based on the appropriate definition of a problem, including the medical, health promotional and health educational aspects, an insight can be gained into the best available solutions to be applied in a specific situation. Health behaviour and actions are nevertheless complex. They form part of a life-style, shaped by interaction between external and personal factors, with medical, health promotional and health educational aspects. Any solution will have to take into consideration these aspects, within a holistic intervention. It should be noted that making analytical distinctions is only a means of learning more about different aspects of a problem, and that all the aspects must be brought together in an intervention.

Medical Solutions

It is important to remind oneself that most medical problems already have medical solutions, taking the form of the prevention, treatment and/or management of health threats and disease. This implies that health education and health promotion can only be considered as complementary and supportive to medical solutions. Unfortunately, there are still a number of medical problems for which there is no medical solution. In this case, the role of health promotion and education is to enable the individuals or populations affected to cope with all the aspects of such a problem, and to help them to mobilize all the support necessary from the medical and social services, as well as from their immediate and wider social environment.

Prevention

When we talk about prevention we mean, in most cases, primary prevention. Different levels of prevention must be taken into consideration, since they will require specific solutions. In general terms, a distinction can be drawn between primary, secondary and tertiary prevention, although there are some other more complex classificatory systems.

1. Primary prevention: This is concerned with preventing the onset of a disease. This implies that it is limited to a 'healthy' population, which could be or is exposed to an unacceptable level of risk from a health threat. Medicine has been the branch of science that has contributed most to our present-day body of knowledge about the causation and spread of a disease. Based on this knowledge, it is possible to define that segment of a population which runs a higher than average risk from a health threat, and which should be included in a preventive intervention. Since external and personal factors, or a combination of both causes disease, preventive interventions will take both into account in the attempt to reduce the risk and protect individuals.

The methods used can include a number of activities. An attempt can be made to eliminate the cause from the environment, as in the case of malaria eradication, prevention of salmonella poisoning, ensuring safe drinking water and reducing air pollution, implementing safety measures at work, prohibiting driving after drinking, isolating the carriers of a disease, etc. In addition, an attempt can be made to raise natural resistance in a person by boosting the immune system through vaccination and immunization, preventing contact with carriers, promoting the use of protective and immunity-enhancing practices, etc. Varied combinations of approaches can be employed, which will affect both the environment and the individual.

Some of these measures can be broadly applied to the whole population, whereas others are appropriate only for a population that is at an unacceptable level of risk from a health threat. In the latter case, it is necessary to define this part of the population at high risk by means of screening programmes, examination of behavioural patterns and general life-styles.

The medical solution, in many cases, will be concerned with the provision of appropriate knowledge about prevention, adequate supplies of preventive materials, provision of adequate services for their implementation, and, in general terms, improving the availability of prevention for the population at risk.

In planning a medical preventive intervention, it is necessary to distinguish between the prevention of disease and the prevention of risk factors. The former is concerned with specific medical causes, whereas the latter is more concerned with prevention of the acquisition of certain types of behaviour, which could increase the risk from a health threat. Examples that occur here include preventing children from experimenting with smoking, encouraging young people to use precautions in their sexual relationships, within the existing social, moral, religious and legal norms, preventing drug abuse, and preventing poor parental practice in raising children.

2. Secondary prevention: This is mainly concerned with the prevention of the further development of existing diseases, or of precursors leading to a disease, involving the control of the situation and the attempt to reverse the processes. In the case of children, secondary prevention will emphasize the early diagnosis and treatment of any disease, and the isolation of the patient, to avoid contact and the spread of that disease throughout the healthy population. Health promotion and education will use medical knowledge to improve people's competence in recognizing the most common diseases and in seeking timely medical help, as well as to enable adults to cope with the management of the disease and the patient.

A new field of activity within the framework of secondary prevention is concerned with people who have been diagnosed as carrying certain genetic traits, which make them prone to certain diseases or which could be activated with certain forms of behaviour. There may be genetic marker, which increases the probability of acquiring a disease such as cystic fibrosis, Alzheimer's disease, etc. or there can be a genetic disposition to cancer, which can be activated through smoking, etc. With growing numbers of discoveries of genetic associations with certain health threats and diseases, and with the possibility of genetic screening being available in the high street, there will be a considerable increase in the awareness about people at risk. The outcome of establishing the presence of a predisposing factor to a health threat (behaviour such as smoking or genetic disposition) can be used to discriminate about features of that population group or set of individuals (insurance, surgery, jobs, child bearing, etc.). These people will require support and counseling as a part of the health promotion and health education activities within secondary prevention.

3. Tertiary prevention: This is concerned with people who have recovered from a disease but who may have some after-effects that restrict their normal life. This may include children who are born with certain handicaps or suffer from the after-effects of a childhood disease; people with infectious diseases, which have turned into chronic states or for which there is no known cure; sufferers from AIDS; cancer patients including terminal cases; and people suffering some disability due to a disease or an accident, as in the case of diabetes. People need to learn how to monitor their state, how to cope with it and how to deal with emergencies. The role of health promotion and education here will be to raise their competence, and enable them to utilize the available support systems.

Treatment

Treatment, as a medical solution usually includes medication, surgical intervention or procedures such as radiation therapy. It can be concerned with the following aspects.

1. Acute episodes: In this instance, the medical profession goes through the process of legitimizing the patient's sick-role, as well as negotiating and implementing some form of treatment. Since such episodes are usually limited in time, since the medical solutions are mostly concerned with medication and other types of medical interventions.

The implications for health promotion and education are numerous: health promotion and health education can influence the kind of information available to the population at risk as well as the general population; and they can influence the decision-making process by making desired decisions more attractive and reducing the fear from negative consequences. Through the evaluation of such processes, it is possible to find out how effective the intervention has been and what needs to be done to remedy any mistakes.

Finally, it should be emphasised that social roles, associated with certain statuses, are governed by norms or expectations, which define the role performance, and may attract sanctions when deviance occurs. For this reason, the role performance of an individual will depend not only on the decision-making process and its outcome, but also on the social support that individual receives in the form of supportive norms, as well as the more general social reinforcement from his/her social environment.

2. Behavioural practices: Numerous behavioural problems can require a medical solution, such as, for example, a whole range of mental illness, which display behavioural symptoms and require medical treatment. There are, however, other behavioural patterns, like those associated with smoking, with obesity, or with hyperactivity in children, which are often interpreted as mundane occurrences, but have also attracted medical solutions.

Management

The health care system is involved in providing services concerned with the management of illness or being at risk. The medical measures concerning management may include provision for the handicapped, mentally ill, chronically ill, etc. Depending on what is required, management needs to cover the at-risk status and the sick role.

1. At-risk status: People may live in areas which are associated with an increased risk from a certain disease, or may be involved in occupations that increase the risk to their health. The management of people with an at-risk status may include protective arrangements in their working environment or protective equipment for personal use. Protection also encompasses the constant monitoring of workers who are exposed to the danger of radiation, or to other noxious substances.

2. Sick role: Once a person has acquired a sick-role, a number of measures will be necessary in managing this status, to enable people to fulfil their sick-role successfully. This includes the post-operative management of patients, as well as the process of rehabilitation.

Health Promotion Solutions

Health promotion solutions will be closely related to the way a problem has been defined in health promotional terms, but will usually include the manipulation of societal factors and the influencing of individual reactions to those factors.

Currently, health promotion activities are based on what is known as the 'Ottawa Charter', signed by the participants of the First International Conference on Health Promotion held in Ottawa in 1986.

The prerequisites for health, according to the Charter, include peace, shelter, education, food, income, a stable ecosystem, sustainable resources, social justice and equity.

There are three main activities related to the fulfillment of these prerequisites. These activities are:

- *Advocacy:* Good health is a major resource for social, economic and personal development, and an important dimension of the quality of life; political, economic, social, cultural, environmental, behavioural and biological factors can all favour good health, or be harmful to it. Health promotion action aims at making these conditions favorable through advocacy for health.

- *Enabling:* Health promotion focuses on achieving equity in health; health promotion action aims at reducing differences in current health status, and ensuring equal opportunities and resources to enable all people to achieve their fullest health potential; this includes a secure foundation in a supportive environment, access to information, life skills and opportunities for making healthy choices. People cannot achieve their fullest health potential unless they are able to take control of those things which determine their health; this must apply equally to women and men.

- *Mediating:* The prerequisites and prospects for health cannot be ensured by the health sector alone; more importantly, health promotion demands co-ordinated action by all concerned: by governments, by health and other social and economic sectors, by non-governmental and voluntary organizations, by local authorities, by industry and by the media; people in all walks of life are involved as individuals, families and communities; professional and social groups and health personnel have a major responsibility to mediate between differing interests in society for the pursuit of health.

Health promotion action means building healthy public policy, creating supportive environments, strengthening community action, developing personal skills and reorienting health services. It is mainly concerned with population or community interventions. It includes a multisectoral approach expressed in multisectoral cooperation.

Environmental interventions

The successful application of a medical solution (including health promotion aspects) requires a conducive and supportive environment (both physical and social).

1. Physical environment: Services available for the solutions of certain health problems make an important contribution to those environmental factors, influencing the success of any intervention. They will depend on 'healthy public policies' as well as the appropriate provision made on an organizational and administrative level. The services to be considered are:

- *Medical services,* which will reflect the type of health care system in the country, including the geographical distribution of hospitals, clinics, GPs, and the proportion of health personnel for a given population.

- *Social services,* which play an important part in helping people to overcome the social effects of their at-risk or sick role; services contribute in the form of professional support, financial support, as well as providing temporary or permanent placement in special institutions.

- *Lay support systems,* are an important form of service structure, usually initiated by individuals or group, which can play a big part in the prevention, management and treatment of diseases; the role of these systems is increasingly recognised as being an effective means of achieving self-reliance and reducing the over-dependence of individuals on the medical system.

2. Social environment: The solution of many problems originating on a societal level requires governmental intervention and community participation in policy planning and execution. This is reflected in the social expectations predominant in the community involved. The type of sanctions will differ, but may have as strong a coercive power as legal or professional sanctions, and may activate strong social support. Norms define the provisions made by the social environment in support of medical solutions. We can differentiate between the following relevant types of norms:

- *Legal norms* - These express the provisions, including rights and duties, defined by law and supported by legal sanctions; legal norms cover a whole range of rights and duties of the individuals, their family, as well as the community in which they live;

- *Professional norms* - These define the rights and duties of members of different profession engaged in the prevention, management or treatment of disease and health risks;

- *Social norms* - These reflect the general culture and value systems of a certain population group or community; they are reflected in individual attitudes to the acceptance and utilization of the services provided.

Individual adjustment

Even when there is a positive and supportive social environment, individuals may still have problems in utilizing or adjusting to its potential. The health promotional activity in this context covers various aspects.

1. Physical environment: Even the presence of positive and supportive norms related to the utilization, compliance and management of a disease might not ensure that individuals might not fully use these services, owing to their perception of existing expectations. This can result in a variety of actions, which when compared with the actual norms, can be expressed in the form of:

- *Conformity* to certain norms, which are perceived to exist, but in fact do not exist, or do not exist in that specific form.

- *Variance,* which goes beyond the accepted limits, or takes harmful forms, in instances where the existing norm is not sufficiently precise.

- *Deviance* from existing expectations or norms, which may occur for many reasons; in some cases, the return to conformity may require, in addition to medical treatment, an increase in social pressure supported by social sanctions.

It is important for planning health promotion interventions to establish whether a certain type of action is the result of a wrong perception of the existing norms or whether the perception corresponds to the existing norms and the type of action is deliberate.

2. Individual reaction to the social environment: This is concerned with the willingness of individuals to participate actively in planning and decision making on a community level. Even where the services do exist, are accessible and available, the general image may be such that people may not want to use them. It may be necessary to change the image or individual perception of that image. The availability of and perceptions attached to the services involved should therefore be explored, with reference to:

- *Medical services,* which for a number of reasons may have a stigma attached to their image, such as cancer hospitals, asylums and clinics for sexually transmitted diseases.

- *Social services,* which may also carry a stigma for certain population groups; quite a large proportion of the population does not take advantage of different kinds of benefits which they are entitled to claim, while there is a problem with the over-utilization of certain social services, resulting in long waiting lists.

- *Lay support systems,* in the form of different self-help groups, which have been in existence for some time, and have provided help and support to a number of people; nevertheless, certain groups of people, for different reasons, do not use this support system, although they could benefit from it, and greater use of existing systems and the creation of additional ones may greatly improve the health of a community.

Health Education Solutions

Given the best social environment and the best medical care available, the health of individuals will still depend on their competence in dealing with the health problems that face them. In order to increase the competence of individuals in dealing with health problems, health education has to address a number of issues.

Knowledge (awareness)

There may be cases where individuals are healthy, and live a long life, without any accurate knowledge about the causes, prevention, treatment and management of certain diseases. This situation is nevertheless rare in industrialized societies, where there is a minimum level of education, and where people are exposed to information through the mass media and want to know the reasons for, as well as the methods of dealing with, a health problem. In this sense, awareness of the existence of a health problem, supported by knowledge about its characteristics, becomes an important aspect of individual competence to deal with it. Health education interventions that are aimed at raising this competence through knowledge will take different forms.

- *Acquisition* of new knowledge, which will depend on the learning process, communication networks and understanding the content; all these aspects need to be taken into account in any health education intervention.

- *Modification* is a more difficult task for health education, since it has to deal with the existing ('false') knowledge and supplement it with new ('accurate') knowledge. This will involve a number of processes, which may include acceptance of innovation, as well as changes in subjective reality based on previously existing knowledge.

- *Operationalisation* means translating existing, accurate knowledge into action. Here health education is dealing with positive resolution of cognitive dissonance, motivation for a positive action, assertion training and acquisition of other social skills, all of that should enhance the probability of a desired action taking place.

Attitudes

If one interprets attitudes as 'internalized social norms', then the general orientation towards a health solution will influence individual attitudes. Various aspects of attitudes are important considerations for health education.

- *Severity:* A health problem must be seen as sufficiently serious or severe to merit a positive action. The perception of severity in health education has been shown to be associated with fear, and is motivational only at an optimal level. If it is too low it may not lead to an action, or if it is too high it may inhibit an action. The question of optimal severity for each specific health threat is of special interest for health education.

- *Susceptibility:* The belief that a person is susceptible to a health threat, "it could happen to me" is an important aspect of a general attitude to a health threat. The feeling of susceptibility is closely related to the problem of the locus of control, and will influence whether an action will take place or not.

- *Utility:* The probability of existing positive knowledge and attitudes resulting in an action will depend on the cost benefit analysis associated with the required action. This will be expressed in terms of the subjective expected utility an individual anticipates from an action, and the anticipated cost involved.

Skills

A number of health actions related to the prevention, treatment and management of a health threat or disease will require a degree of competence in specific skills to cope with the problem. The role of health education is to enable individuals to learn those skills, and to achieve this it will be necessary to utilise the following concepts:

- *Communication and learning:* The process of communication is very complex, and its analysis includes a number of approaches, from which that most appropriate for a specific problem will have to be selected. Variation also applies to the learning capacity of individuals, and the learning processes, which will have to be activated to achieve the best possible results.

- *Coping and modification:* In certain cases, modification of knowledge, attitudes or behaviour may produce the desired results. In other cases, when this is not possible, the individuals will have to learn to cope with the existing problem in terms of management and coming to terms with the unavoidable outcome. The role of health education in this area is very important and needs to be developed further.

- *Decision-making and operationalisation:* The ultimate aim of most health education interventions is for an individual to operationalise the accurate knowledge, the positive attitudes and the acquired skills in terms of an action aimed at the prevention, treatment or management of a disease. Health education has a role in providing the necessary cues, which will trigger off a desired action.

- *Competence:* The recent shift of emphasis from risk factors to healthy life-styles and the emphasis on self-reliance has required a new approach in health education. Its aim has been to raise the general 'competence' of individuals to look after their health and not be too dependent on the health care system. In this sense, health education is a part of general education for life and survival, as well as for taking on the responsibility for the improvement of one's own quality of life. There are various programmes concerned with improving a person's competence, and a variety of technologies that enable people to carry out a more accurate diagnosis or to be able to monitor their health and to discover any early signs of increased risk from a health threat. People may be encouraged to acquire scales to measure their weight; there are simple-to-operate gadgets to measure blood pressure and levels of blood cholesterol; there is a simple test to check on blood sugar, equipment to monitor one's biorhythm and alpha waves, and even a do-it-yourself acupuncture kit. All kinds of equipment for exercising at home (stationary bicycles, rowing machines, weight lifting equipment, mobile running tracks, etc.) are commercially available. Videotapes are a very popular technological development with programmes covering practically every aspect of health. There are regular television and radio programmes concerned with health issues. All these developments have resulted in an increase in people's competence and willingness to accept responsibility for their own health, and to improve their ability to deal with health issues in the privacy of their home. For people who feel the need to improve their competence, a popular way is either to establish or join a self-help group. Many such groups exist; some of them are highly successful and have been popular for a long time. This form of social support has been found to be very valuable in maintaining certain health-enhancing behavioural patterns such as not smoking, dieting, and controlling drug intake or alcohol abuse.

Chapter 4

INTERVENTIONS

Introduction
Health Promotion Intervention
Health Education Intervention

Health promotion and health education in a setting and a 'health promoting setting' differ, and this affects the planning and carrying out of a number of interventions to bring the activity from an administrative to a consumer level.

Planning interventions for a 'health promoting setting' will follow the steps of the general planning process, which include:

- Definition of the problem/s in terms of health promotion and health education; this should include establishing people's needs and base line data as a part of the assessment process;

- Carrying out the planning (short and long term); role distribution; commitment, including impact assessment based on simulation methods;

- Definition of aims and objectives based on the choice of appropriate solutions;

- Provision of resources (personnel and finances);

- Monitoring the process through quality management;

- Evaluation and audit.

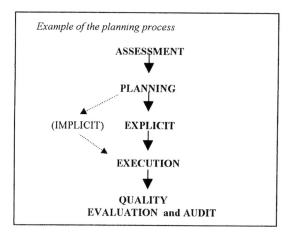

Example of the planning process

ASSESSMENT

PLANNING

(IMPLICIT)   EXPLICIT

EXECUTION

QUALITY
EVALUATION and AUDIT

A difference can be drawn between implicit and explicit planning. It can be assumed that health promotion and health education in a family setting will be subject to an 'implicit' planning process and that parents will 'do what is normal' in bringing up their children. The interpretation of 'normal' will be reflected in adults' normative behaviour according to the social norms or expectations about bringing up a child. The family household as a setting may also be exposed to a health promotion and health education intervention from outside, which will be subject to 'explicit' planning. Such a planned intervention usually starts with an assessment including a number of questions that need to be answered before any planning can take place. These are discussed in the Chapter 6 of this book.

In the case of a 'health promoting setting' such as a city, hospital, general practice, school, enterprise, etc., planning will be explicit and will demonstrate all the characteristics of a formal planning process.

One of the main principles of any 'health promoting setting' is that it should be composed of 'health promoting units'. An example is a 'health promoting city', which at present is known as a 'healthy city'. The difference lies in the approach used in planning and execution of HP/HE interventions as illustrated in the following diagram:

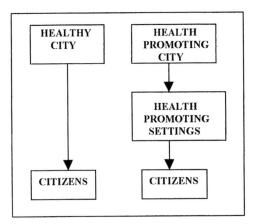

At present there are over a thousand healthy cities throughout the world and nearly all of them operate mainly on the administrative level with a number of specific interventions carried out for the benefit of their citizens. The 'health promoting city' is characterised by the 'health promoting settings' through which it reaches the citizens. These 'health promoting settings' (hospitals, schools, enterprises, etc.) plan and execute HP/HE interventions within the sphere of their competence and activities.

Within the framework of a systems approach, the planning unit can be the city as a whole or certain institutions within a city such as hospitals, schools, enterprises, etc. It does not really matter whether the starting point is the city or an institution in the city, the whole system will be encompassed in the end. If one starts from a hospital, the commitment to include outreach into the community will ultimately require that the hospital initiates the changes in the city as a whole. The same applies if one starts from a 'healthy city', which will need to initiate the change of the status of its institutions and motivate them to become 'health promoting settings'.

Health promotion deals with external factors arising from the physical and social environment. Interventions should be planned to solve the problems established through the assessment process and could include the improvement of the living conditions of the general population, as well as of certain high-risk groups. It is based on an understanding of the medical, social and political aspects of the problems and their solutions.

In terms of the planning process it is necessary to differentiate planning on the administrative and the consumer levels. Within a 'healthy city' for example, the planning will include the transformation of the local institutions into 'health promoting settings', whereas in a setting within a city (hospital, school, etc.) the planning will be concerned with interventions on a consumer level.

Choice of topics

In the case of planning interventions related to health promotion on the consumer level, the focus on topics will be based on the problems established as a result of the assessment of the setting. They may include:

- *a disease* entity, a disease complex, or a level of health can be used in measurement; they can be measured in terms of incidence and prevalence, distribution, causation, prevention, treatment, management and outcome;

- *a process*, which can include the stages of becoming ill; awareness of the problem; competence of dealing with it; communication with the social environment; coping, decision-making, learning, etc.;

- *a structure*, which will include the organization of the external, as well as the internal system within which the intervention is taking place; power structure; role distribution; networks, etc;

- *a model*, which will include the development or testing of a scientifically supported model of the system within which the intervention is taking place; the theories linking the parts of the model; the instruments applied for measurement, etc;

- *a population group*, which could represent the whole or a part of the population affected by the activities of the setting; it may be the population of a community or an institution; it could also include specific target populations defined by age, sex, occupation, people with specific lifestyles and/or behavioural patterns, educational level, competence and their potential to participate in the change process;

- *a relationship*, which could include the existing relationship frameworks, such as doctor-patient, mother-child, manager-worker, teacher-pupil, etc;

- *a social institution*, which could also be defined as a setting, such as hospital, school, family, workplace, etc;

- *a discrete action*, which could be an immunization or a screening programme, improvement of physical environment, a behaviour modification clinic, etc;

- *a network analysis*, which could include the study of the existing professional, social, administrative, kin and other types of networks.

Any of the above mentioned topics or a combination of several of them can be the subject matter of a health promotion and health education intervention. In each case, the planner should be able to answer the following questions:

- What are the characteristics of the setting?
- Why this particular topic?
- What is already known or has been done/written about that topic?
- What does the intervention hope and plan to achieve (aims)?
- How can the achievements be assessed?

These questions require that consideration should be given to a number of issues, such as the existing expertise, the opportunity of acquiring expert support, the time and money available and the expectations of the stakeholders. Some topics lend themselves to a clear description of the intervention in terms of aims and objectives, which subsequently allows for the use of relevant analysis of data and an objective statement of consequences. There are, however, some topics that are relatively vague and where only descriptive inferences will be justified. Depending on its topic, the intervention can be defined in terms of its feasibility and expected outcomes.

One of the first steps after choosing a topic is to identify a baseline related to that topic. This serves a double purpose: it provides a basis from which the effects of an intervention can be measured, and it indicates the most relevant problem areas to be tackled by an intervention. Very often the selected topic is related to the needs of the target population. This requires the examination and definition of those needs and the establishment of the difference between the needs and the wishes of the target population. In some cases, the health needs may be latent or of secondary importance, compared to the more generally felt needs such as poverty, bereavement, paying for an imminent wedding or an unwanted pregnancy. If health promotion and health education need to deal with such crises, this will have to be taken into account in the planning process, since it will not be easy to concentrate the attention of the target population on some health needs which may at the time be considered as unimportant or irrelevant. The establishment of needs can be carried out objectively (externally) by using professional judgement and the preferences of the stakeholders, or subjectively, by using the opinions of the target population.

Definition of specific aims

Given the definition of a health problem in medical terms, with special reference to the intervention required on a societal and a personal level, the description of specific aims of the health promotion aspect of the intervention will cover the following areas:

Physical and social environment

The physical environment may need improvement to provide people with the possibility of remaining healthy. Similarly, the social environment may require the modification of social norms as well as of the individual's perceptions, in order to enhance the prevailing chances of survival and improvements in health. Depending on the existing situation, the aims of a health promotion intervention take the following points into account:

- *the physical environment* - the aim could be to remove any health hazards, and improve living and working conditions in an area;

- *social norms* - the aim could be to modify or reinforce existing norms or create new ones according to whether or not they are conducive to health;

- *the perception of norms* - the aim could be to change or reinforce individual perception of norms, since individuals may perceive that there are norms when no norms in fact exist, or they may wrongly perceive sanctions associated with norms.

Community services and lay support systems

The aims of a health promotion intervention may be concerned with the improvement of existing services and the provision of support from self-help groups. Specific aims can, therefore, target:

- *community services* - the aim could be to improve or reinforce existing services or to create new ones, including health as well as social services, depending on whether they are conducive to health and satisfy the needs of the community;

- *lay support systems* - the aim could be to support existing or help in developing new lay support systems in the form of self-help groups, according to the character of the health problem and the needs of the community.

Definition of objectives

The way the chosen aim or aims will be realized can be expressed in terms of the objectives of the intervention. These can be derived from the findings as a result of the simulation approach, which may include several options, expressed in different scenarios. These may include:

Physical environment

The definition of the problem, and the choice of the solutions with regard to the physical environment, as part of the objectives of the planned intervention.

Social environment (norms)

Depending on the chosen aim, the objectives could include the creation of new norms or the reinforcement and improvement of existing norms, as well as the modification of individual perceptions of norms. These include:

- *social norms* - the objectives could be concerned with creating new norms, and reinforcing or changing existing norms; in addition to changing norms, the objectives could also be differentiated depending on whether the norms in question are general or specific; the objectives of the intervention could also be specified according to which of the following aspects of a norm needs to be modified: legitimization, coercive power and/or social support;

- *perception of norms* - the norms can only be as effective as people perceive them to be and if they accept and conform to them; the objectives could, therefore, also include the changing or reinforcing of individual perception of a norm, and its specific characteristics.

Services

The achievement of separate aims will each require a different set of specific objectives, such as:

- *community services* - the objectives may include the reinforcement and improvement of existing services or the creation of new community services according to the needs of the population; they may also include improvements in the accessibility and attractiveness of the services in order to improve utilisation and compliance within the community;

- *lay support systems* - the objectives may include specific measures for financial and/or expert support for the existing lay support systems, or they may initiate the creation of new lay support groups in the form of self-help groups.

Methods

The achievement of objectives will require the choice of a combination of appropriate methods. These will mainly be concerned with the manipulation of, and individual adjustment to, external factors. Any change will depend on a combination of health promotion and health education approaches, but here we are mainly concerned with the former. The most commonly used methods include:

Advocacy

This concept defines the role of the health promotion agents (bearing in mind the multisectoral approach) as advocates for the rights and need-satisfaction of a population or group. Agents can fulfil this role either within the system (for example, by being 'advocate-planners') or by placing themselves outside the system (as for example some pressure groups, community workers who work outside the system through pressure groups). In either case, advocacy is an important part of a health promotion intervention.

Mass media

The mass media approach can be extremely effective in changing social norms or expectations, as well as in changing people's perceptions of these norms. It is also successful in transmitting information about health threats or diseases, and the availability of relevant services, including the existence of new formal or lay services. The following aspects are important in using mass media:

- *the source*, of the message will influence its credibility;

- *the message*, which will be most effective if it is composed with clarity, with the right appeal, using the appropriate language, showing relevance to the reader and providing the reader with an acceptable solution (who, what, when, where, how?);

- *the medium*, which should be easily accessible to people and form a part of their usual means of acquiring information on a variety of subjects;

- *the legitimising agent*, who should participate in any mass media campaign, and reinforce the message either publicly or on a person-to-person level.

Community organization

Community organization, as a means of ensuring community participation in the prevention, management and treatment of disease, will be useful in the creation, improvement and management of services in a community. Communities may be faced with three kinds of problems, each of which will require a specific approach:

- *problems communities themselves can solve*, which will require the mobilisation of community resources and the active participation of community members;

- *problems which communities can solve only with outside help*, which implies that community resources are not sufficient, and outside help in expertise or resources will be required;

- *problems that require outside help*, where the community members need to have the knowledge and skills for mobilizing this help, and which will usually include a multisectoral co-ordination of efforts and resources.

Indicators

Any evaluation of the achievement of the aims and objectives of a health promotion intervention will require a definition of appropriate indicators. Some of the important indicators are set out below.

Changes in the physical environment

Diagnosing the problem within a physical environment will provide the basis for the selection of appropriate indicators such as a reduction in unemployment, or air pollution, an improvement in transport and communications, or the setting up of services.

Changes in norms and their perception

Any change concerning norms is a social process, and will require social indicators, whereas the changes in personal perceptions of norms should be measured by surveying the individuals in a population. Both types of measurement should use indicators that are sensitive enough to measure the changes in the following aspects of norms and their perception:

- *content* of a norm in relation to a health threat or disease, and the expectations concerning people's behaviour and action;

- *specificity* of the level of expectations which will be needed to assess people's behaviour in terms of conformity, variance and deviance;

- *prevalence* or awareness of the existence of a norm in a population or a specific population group;

- *coercive power* of a norm in terms of sanctions related to the deviant behaviour;

- *legitimisation* of the expectations by the professions and important others;

- *social support* that can be expected from the immediate and wider social environment for conformist behaviour.

Utilisation of services and self-help groups

Many indicators have been developed for the measurement of the utilisation of services, which are also useful in evaluating a health promotion intervention. Additional indicators may be required to measure the effectiveness of community participation in such areas as the planning and management of existing services, the creation of new services, the level of self-reliance in a community, and the changes following a health promotion intervention.

- *Services:* In addition to standardized indicators for the measurement of the utilisation of services, new indicators need to be developed which enable existing or newly created social mechanisms, in order to identify or prevent community participation in the planning and management of services.

- *Self-help:* Since there is no standardized way of measuring the social process involved in the development of self-help movements in a community, new indicators are necessary. These include: the measurement of the existing levels of self-reliance and self-help in a community in general, and specifically for the problem relevant to the health promotion intervention in question; the community need for social support in general, and specifically in relation to the health issue in question; and the changes achieved by the health promotion intervention.

Criteria

The term 'criteria' refers to the units that are used in the measurement of the contribution of a certain objective to the achievement of a specified aim. They also include a value judgement about a measured level of achievement. On a population level, a planner may, for example, be faced with making the following decisions.

- How to measure the different *aspects* of awareness within a population in order to establish which are contributing most to an activity, and which through their absence are associated with non-activity.

- How to measure the different *levels* of different aspects of awareness in order to establish the optimal, compared to the minimal or maximal level, which can then be used as a measure of success or failure.

- How to choose the *target population* for such measurements in terms of relevance, accessibility and representativeness, for the study population.

- How to measure the *prevalence* of the expected action, accepting the limitations of reported as compared to observed behaviour, and the problems of the validity and reliability of the collected information.

Instruments

Once the indicators have been chosen and the criteria for their measurement and assessment have been agreed upon, the planner will have to translate them into instruments, which will then be used for the collection of desired information.

There is a whole set of different forms that such instruments can take, from structured questionnaires and the 'aide memoir' to diaries and scaling methods. Instruments are differentiated according to whether their purpose is to produce qualitative or quantitative data.

The value judgement about the expected levels of change, as compared with those observed, will be important for the analysis and for justifiable inferences. The instruments should be tested for validity and reliability.

Resources

The resources necessary for a health promotion intervention will vary in kind and origin. Since any health promotion intervention is by definition dependent upon multisectoral co-ordination and cooperation, the resources will originate from different institutions and government bodies. The kinds of resources required are:

Financial

Any improvements in the physical environment will be dependent upon the available financial support. The level of support has to be taken into account when planning an intervention, and can be expanded by community participation in the planning process. Health promotion also involves the use of mass media, which are, in most cases, commercially run and very expensive. It is, therefore, necessary to make provisions for covering the expenses of the production and publication of messages via mass media. Since these and other similar activities require professional expertise, financial support may be needed for consultancy. Evaluation, which may include population surveys, will also require funding.

Material

The preparation and publication of material to be distributed in different forms will have to be carried out by experts, since the population is exposed to a high level of professionalism in advertising and public relation products in their everyday life. In addition to technical experts, it will be necessary to plan for communication experts to be involved in the choice and formulation of the messages.

Monitoring and Evaluation

Evaluation of any health promotion intervention should be a part of the wider approach to accountability, which includes assessment, quality management, evaluation and audit. (For detailed description of these processes see Chapter 6 in this book).

Health education, in its reduced scope since the introduction of health promotion, now deals mainly with personal and small group factors. It should still be recognized as the necessary and complementary aspect to health promotion for any intervention aimed at improving the health of a population.

Differential diagnosis

Once the base-line information has been collected by means of the assessment process, the problem is how to translate it into a health education intervention. For this purpose, it will be necessary to work out a system for utilising each different kind of information collected. This can be helped by 'differential diagnosis', which draws on the idea of a passage through the cause-effect system of the individual or group in question. By a process of elimination, it is possible to arrive at the factors that seem to be the most promising for the achievement of the set aims, and to develop an indicator set, which will include the domains relevant for the achievement of the aims.

The information collected can only be operationalised for health education purposes if each domain of information is examined separately to see how it can contribute to planning an intervention. Each domain will provide a general picture of the relevant factors contributing to the improvement of competence, if that is the aim of the study, while differential diagnosis will help in selecting those which are likely to be affected by a health education intervention. A value judgement must be made about the minimal and optimal needs affecting competence, given constraints of the social environment and the capabilities of the individual or group in question.

According to the kind of information collected, two main types of factors can be distinguished: enabling factors and contributing factors. Plans for intervention can be developed in relation to these factors. The established needs of the members of the population and the available opportunities and resources at their disposal need also to be taken into account.

Enabling factors

Enabling factors are considered to be those which contribute to the provision of an environment, within which individuals or groups live which are conducive to health. This environment can best be described by a set of variables, as set out below:

- *Location* – including type of settlement, amenities, neighborhood, dwellings, climatic conditions and available space in the dwelling;

- *Economy* – including the general economic state of a country, the income per capita, the level of technological development, source of income, employment, migration, resources for health care;

- *Social organization* – including the political system, the degree of governmental and social responsibility; social stratification; political organization and the participation of the population in deciding about their own destiny and in solving existing national and local problems.

- *Communications* – including the possibility of mobility and travel, which will enhance personal exchanges; the network of a media communication system, which would include film, radio, T.V., video, and the press as well as telephone, cable and information technology; the organisational network, which would include meetings, gatherings and visits; personal communication systems (including access by transport systems to kin and social networks) and access to the existing means of communication, such as telephone and electronic communication;

- *Value systems* – including prevalent religious beliefs, which reflect one aspect of the existing value system and can have an important influence on a number of health issues.

- *Education* – including simple differentiation between levels of education, such as functional illiteracy, basic (primary), secondary and higher education; there is a direct relationship between the level of education and the health state of an individual or a family.

- *State of health* – including the situation as expressed as the prevalent morbidity and mortality patterns, which will influence the intervention aims.

- *Health care* – including the existing health care system available to the population and different population groups.

Contributing factors

Within a specific physical and social environment, different individuals and groups (such as the family) develop different ways of adjusting to the environment and will manifest different patterns of utilization of available resources. Therefore, it is possible to differentiate between individuals and groups in terms of their social characteristics, which can directly affect their state of health and their ability to cope with different health problems. Different individual and group characteristics, which in turn influence the state of health of members, are strongly influenced by external conditions. To explore individual and group characteristics, it is valuable to relate the information about these characteristics to the information collected about the external environment. This makes it possible to establish which kinds of opportunities are offered by the society and how individuals and groups utilize them. The most important contributing factors are:

- *Residence*- includes the type of residence; this will reflect geographical characteristics as well as the socio-cultural and economic position; it will also reflect the available means of communication, mobility and transportation; residence can be classified as urban or rural and as optimal/adequate/poor.

- *Mobility* – includes measures of the amount of time people have been living in a certain community; it can be assumed that an immigrant individual or group, living a short time in a community and with relatively limited access to social support, will need a higher level of competence to deal with health problems than an individual or group living a long time in a community and able to mobilize social support in a crisis situation.

- *Housing* – includes the circumstances in which h an individual or group lives and brings up children; it can be classified as optimal/adequate/poor, according to the number of rooms per person, the placement of amenities and the type of existing protection against the elements, pests, insects, vermin, dampness, etc.

- *Subsistence* – includes indicators of the wealth of an individual or a family, classified as wealthy, adequate and poor, depending on the source of income, the number of economically active members and the amount of property they possess.

- *Domestic group* – includes descriptions of the immediate environment into which a child is born and can take many different forms and includes: a number of people with different relationships; the number of generations living together, the kin relationships of the members of the domestic group, the cycle of individual and group development and the type of conjugal roles within the domestic group.

- *Networks* – includes the possibility of mobilizing resources through kinship or friendship networks; the differentiation of networks can be made on two levels: the extent of individual and group and friendship networks and the quality of relationship within those networks.

- *Education* – includes the recognition that the members of a family will have different orientations towards health problems and their solutions according to their educational level; two types of orientation should be distinguished for health education purposes: cosmopolitan and parochial. The former will include families with a higher level of education and a more scientific approach to health problems, while the latter will include families with basic education whose interpretation of health problems will depend on opinions of relatives, friends and the popular local press;

- *Social position* – includes the implications of the type of the social structure of a society, according to which its members will occupy different social positions; this social stratification, in terms of social class, status, caste, etc., differentiates a person's position on a social scale, which for the purpose of health education interventions can be divided into at least three levels (with a possible transitional category): high, moderate and low. The allocation of a social position is determined by occupation, type of work and status within the organization, as well as by gender and marital status.

- *Values and norms* – include the recognition that every society has its general value system, variously interpreted within different domestic groups. In addition to differences in their perception of values, domestic groups may also be differentiated according to the level of adherence to social norms, reflecting the existing value system

- *State of health* – includes the recognition that the type and frequency of health problems met by a domestic group depends on the general state of health of its members. The state of health will also influence the need for and means of utilization of available health services.

Personal characteristics

The position of an individual in the society can be explored by using the same questions as for group characteristics.

There are, however, a number of additional characteristics, which are specific to the individual. These are concerned with the individual's genetic make-up, personality, opinions, feelings, intentions, competencies, etc.

Since most of these characteristics are represented by concepts, which are theoretical constructs, their measurement will depend on the development of specific tests. Theoretical constructs refer to concepts such as intelligence, experience of stress, aptitude, etc. They are not taken to be self-evident, as are, for example, characteristics such as height, weight, sex and age, and need to be carefully defined before they can be measured. The individual characteristics necessary for a differential diagnosis depend on the aims of the intervention and should be selected with a view to the overall framework of health promotion and health education methods.

The planning process

Once a topic has been chosen, based on the existing situation, derived from the assessment process and the needs of the target population, the intervention will follow the normal steps of a planning process. These steps, in summary, include the definition of aims, establishment of objectives or the ways these aims will be achieved, choice of indicators and criteria for the assessment of processes and outcomes:

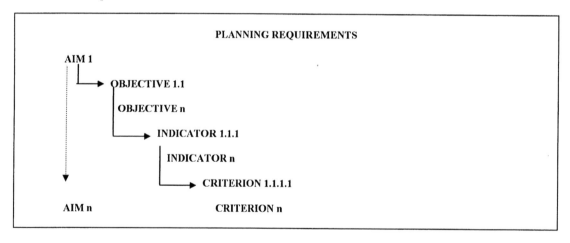

One can differentiate between the short-term and the long-term planning process. The short-term planning process addresses an acute situation and is expected to produce an immediate outcome. The long-term planning process is usually part of a continuous effort of improving the health of a population and may include a number of short-term programmes. The outcome in this case will be cumulative and may be postponed for a number of years before it is clearly visible.

Depending on the problem, planning needs to differentiate between the health promotion and health education aspects of the intervention and will have to take into account the characteristics as well as potential of each aspect of the intervention.

Definition of specific aims

Once the problem has been defined in medical terms, namely the identification of the specific medical actions required for the protection and improvement of health, or the prevention or management of a disease, it is possible to carry out an educational diagnosis and define the aims of a health education intervention. These may include:

- *Knowledge* - The aims can be to increase, correct or improve the existing knowledge or lack of it concerning a health threat or disease, and the available solutions in terms of prevention, management or treatment of that specific health problem.

- *Attitudes* - It still seems to be accepted that, in general, attitudes can enhance or inhibit a health action or behaviour modification; it is, however, doubtful whether changes in attitudes will always result in changes of behaviour. The aims could, therefore, include the acquisition of positive attitudes, or a positive way of resolving cognitive dissonance if attitudes cannot be changed.

- *Skills* - Behaviour modification usually depends on the skills required to manage the transitional period, and to establish new behavioural patterns. Skills are also required in coping with new situations (childbirth, bereavement, unemployment, divorce etc.), and form an important part of a health education intervention. The aims of health education must take these required skills into consideration when trying to achieve self-reliance and competence in the improvement of personal and family health.

Definition of objectives

The achievement of aims will depend on the setting of appropriate objectives. Concerning knowledge, attitudes and skills, these can be differentiated in terms of the following processes:

- *Acquisition* – Specific descriptions are required of the objectives that will be most promising for the development of the knowledge, desirable attitudes and necessary skills required for improvements in health. Each of the three aims mentioned will require different objectives concerning the processes involved and methods used;

- *Modification* - The set of objectives needed to achieve the modification of existing knowledge, attitudes or skills will have to take into account the approaches and methods which have been shown to be effective in achieving such a change.

Methods

Depending on their aims and objectives, health education interventions have a range of different methods at their disposal:

- *Information* - The transmission and acquisition of information is associated with the knowledge necessary for the awareness of a threat, and the availability of ways to prevent it. The methods used include mass media, public lectures, group work and individual advice. The theories which explain the relevance of an approach include learning and communication theories, advertising and market research.

- *Counselling* - To enable individuals to cope with a health problem in terms of behaviour modification, the adjustment of their subjective reality, the desired role performance and a general increase in their personal competence, they may require intensive support in the form of counselling. This can take a variety of forms appropriate to the individual's needs and capacities;

- *Group work* - Changes in attitudes, as well as ability to cope with certain emotional problems, may require a supportive environment, which can either be found in a family or in a group of a specific kind. It has been found that group dynamics can be conducive to changes in attitudes, the resolution of cognitive dissonance, changes in self-esteem, improving self-assertion, and readjusting the perceived locus of control. Groups are also helpful in accepting commitments through negotiation and group pressure.

Indicators, criteria, instruments

The aims and objectives should be defined in such a way that they can be measured in terms of the initial situation and the subsequent changes:

- *Specific indicators* - It is recognized that when the aim is an improvement in health by means of changing a life-style, it may be difficult to select specific indicators which could monitor and record such a change. It will be necessary to define a life-style as a system, decide on the relevant factors within that system and then plan an evaluation of changes within these factors or in their interrelationship.

- *Criteria for optimal change* - Most behaviour associated with an increased risk from a disease or a health threat is a necessary part of everyday life and survival (eating, exercise, sex, etc.), and only a few are optional and represent acquired habits (alcohol, smoking, etc.). Any evaluation of a health education intervention will have to define the criteria in terms of the 'minimal' and 'optimal' degree of change required for the prevention, management and treatment of a disease.

Instruments

Population studies use questionnaires for the collection of information, which can then be translated into quantitative data. It should be appreciated that qualitative data can provide a better insight into the more subtle changes which follow a health education intervention, in addition to the more obvious measurable changes in overt behaviour. The instruments developed for the exploration of indicators and criteria can, therefore, range from postal questionnaires to in-depth case studies.

Resources

The new concept of health education as an intensive and personal intervention, requires greater resources in terms of money, time and personnel.

- *Financial* - Financial support is required for the establishment and maintenance of supportive services required by individuals, for the cost of educational programmes, and for monitoring and evaluating the interventions.

- *Material* - Material resources will include the provision of special premises and means of transport, educational material for schools and inservice training programmes, for special educational programmes concerning new health threats and for new educational and information technology.

- *Personnel* – Health educational work with individuals is labour intensive, and will require a great number of educators; health educational and health promotional work with groups and populations, using a multi-sectoral approach, will require additional in-service training and expertise in monitoring and evaluating planned interventions.

Monitoring and evaluation

It is not possible to envisage an intensive personal intervention of a professional standard, without monitoring the process through quality management and evaluating the outcomes. The criteria will include the level of benefit for the clients, and professional responsibility will be expressed in the avoidance of any unforeseen negative side effects (for detailed description see Chapter 6 in this book).

Chapter 5

INTERVENTION METHODS

Introduction
Personal Approach
Group Approach
Community Approach
Mass Media Approach

This section deals with the methods available and currently in use for the purpose of a health promotion and health education intervention (Baric, 1990). The methods presented should be considered within the general framework of the settings approach. They should form a part of the impact assessment process, using simulation methods, which should include various scenarios. The methods chosen should represent the optimal outcome derived from simulation processes.

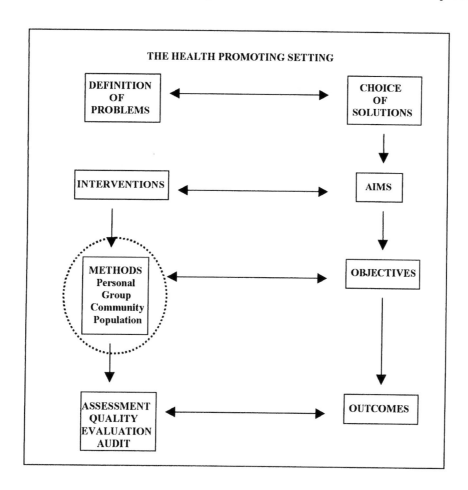

The choice of HP/HE methods will depend on the definition of the problem and the choice of appropriate solution. Within that solution, the aim will be to mount an intervention and the objectives will include the appropriate methods. A health promoting setting is assumed to have a quality management system, which will be used to monitor the processes, whereas evaluation will assess the outcome of the intervention.

The differentiation of methods according to different models has become obsolete, for a number of reasons, two of which are most important. The first one is the total discreditation of the notion of HP/HE "models". Most of the models used in the past did not conform to the so called reality, because they were merely expressed as a number of boxes, indicating parts of the model, linked with arrows, defining the relationship between the boxes. In reality the arrows did not represent anything. What happened was that the author would invent a system with a number of parts (boxes), without bothering to test the theories, defining the relationships among the parts (arrows linking the boxes).

Another reason for inadequacy of models is that owing to recent developments in information technology, the transmission of information, which was usually limited to specific individuals or groups (verbally or through the media), has been replaced by wide ranging access to information, which has not only increased individual knowledge, but also globally influenced the value systems and social expectations (norms). The Internet has expanded the boundaries of the 'global village' and people express 'neighbourly' concerns for people, of whose existence a few years ago they were completely ignorant.

Because of this blurring of boundaries between the effects of different communication methods and the lack of scientific basis for previous models, the notion of specific models has largely been abandoned, and each method with its own potential is considered to be part of a more general or 'ecological' approach. Within this general approach, it is possible to differentiate between the personal, group, community and population (mass media) methods, and to consider their applications in HP/HE interventions within the new settings. The choice of the right mix of methods will depend on a differential diagnosis of the problem and the outcome of simulation procedures. In a systems framework the question is not which method to use, but amongst all the methods used, which should be given the greatest emphasis and most of the available resources, at what time and for which segment of the population.

Methods differ according to the status of the agents involved. Informal agents (such as some health education and health promotion officers, health journalists) can influence the clients indirectly, either through the mass media or through some mediators with a professional status. Parents, as a special case, will use methods involved in bringing up children, which are considered to be a part of the socialization process of the child. Formal agents (such as doctors, teachers, or some health promotion officers) will use methods that enable them to interact with clients directly on a one-to-one or group basis. The professional status of the latter category of agents should ensure the protection of clients' interests and rights.

The expected outcome of a health promotion or health education intervention is the health gain of the clients. This is often dependent on the clients' health behaviour, which will affect their state of health. There is a difference between health-related and health-directed behaviour. Health-*related* behaviour includes any behaviour or action that can affect a person's health. The person may not be aware that a particular form of behaviour is affecting his/her health or may not be motivated by that knowledge. In general, it can be said that any human behaviour (for whatever purpose) can be health-related. Health-*directed* behaviour is considered to be aimed consciously and intentionally at the promotion of one's health and the avoidance of risks or illnesses.

Another important difference can be drawn between 'normative' behaviour and the decisions based on choices. Most human behaviour is *normative*, in the sense that people conform to norms or the expectations current in their social environment. These kinds of behaviour are treated as 'normal' and people act without any explicit decision-making processes. An example of this kind of behaviour is getting dressed in the morning. The norm is to be clothed in public and the action is 'automatic', 'routine' or 'normal'. The examination of people's behaviour within a normative framework is very important for the planning of health promotion and health education interventions. These will have different aims according to whether behaviour is 'conformist' or 'deviant', according to the relevant social expectations or norms. In addition to the concepts of conformity and deviance, the concept of 'variance' is useful. This implies that although behaviour may not exactly fit social expectations (norms), if it is still within the limits of tolerance, it should be treated as 'variant' behaviour. For example, the norm is not to walk naked in public, and a dressed person would be considered as 'conformist'. There is, however, a considerable tolerance in the 'variance' of the interpretation of the term 'dressed', especially with regard to footwear. When going to a wedding, a person with socks and shoes would be a conformist, a person with sandals and no socks could be considered a 'variant' and a bare-footed person could be considered a deviant. The labeling of course depends on the context in which the behaviour is taking place. These concepts are very important for health promotion and health education interventions since there are different acceptable ways of dealing with each of them. Societies have the well-defined ways of dealing with deviants, according to norms associated with a specific behaviour, while ways of dealing with variants are less well defined.

New problems, which emerge as the result of new knowledge and experience, may not as yet be regulated by norms so that behaviour associated with them is the result of the *decision-making* process. In the absence of social expectations (norms), a person makes a choice about the required action, based on a prediction about the utility of the outcome and the probability of achieving such an outcome. The choice of an action depends on the available alternatives, assessed according to preferences in the light of existing constraints. Rationality here replaces normative behaviour.

The right mix of methods for the HP/HE intervention appropriate to the status of the agent, the characteristics of the setting, the outcome of the differential diagnosis of the problem and the selection of solutions, should result in the health gain of a client.

Each of the available methods has certain advantages and disadvantages:

- *The personal approach* – has the advantage of utilizing a differential diagnosis of the individual's problems, addressing personal needs and providing direct help; on the other hand the in-depth analysis as a part of the differential diagnosis may be carried out by amateurs and not professionals in the field of behavioural sciences, which may vitiate the approach.

- *The group approach* – has the advantage of being able to change people's attitudes; the disadvantage here lies in creating dependency among members on the group, thus activating group mechanisms which can be difficult to control;

- *The community participation approach* – has the advantage that the community members can take over the responsibility for their actions; the disadvantage lies in the application of this approach in situations where there are no communities in the HP/HE sense, but only groups of people sharing the same location;

- *The population (mass media) approach* – has the advantage of reaching large segments of the population simultaneously, which is important for changing norms; the disadvantage lies in the possibility of distributing information that may not be appropriate for certain segments of the population.

The methods used in HP/HE interventions are supported by theories, which explain why and how they should work. In following sections these theories are presented within the framework of each specific approach .

Introduction

There are many situations where an intervention will require a personal approach depending on the needs of the clients and the capabilities of the agents. The personal approach should be in the hands of agents with a professional status, which should guarantee the protection of a client's rights. Since HP/HE activities do not have a fully professional status, the agents will be bound by the professional status they bring into the interaction (for example, as doctors, teachers, nurses, social workers, psychologists, or trainers).

In the personal approach, the *medical* definition of a problem should provide information about the relevant risk factors and health threats, their characteristics, and the means of prevention, management and treatment on an individual level.

The *health promotional* definition should include information about the environmental factors (such as social expectations or norms), necessary to influence individual actions concerning health protection and improvement, as well as the description of any mechanisms that enable individuals to influence and change their physical and social environment.

The *health educational* definition should indicate the areas of improvement necessary for possible modification of an individual's normative behaviour, in decision-making and taking action.

The outcome of these definitions influences the choice of methods and contents. Within the personal approach the most important processes are: learning, communicating, decision making, socialisation, interviewing and counselling.

Learning

Education is being both a most important growth industry, labour intensive and attracting large capital investments from a whole array of sources. Its importance has been appreciated for a long time, and it has generated many research and development projects. The underlying concern has been to understand the ways in which people learn, to improve upon them and draw on the most effective and efficient methods of teaching. Since a learning situation mainly involves a person's interaction with other people, communication is recognized as an important aspect of learning.

Most health education interventions are based on an explicit or implicit theory (Jehu, 1967), which provides the rationale for the chosen approach, and explains the processes involved and the expected outcomes. Most 'cognitive' health education models are based on some aspects of particular learning theories, and utilize them in carrying out a health education intervention. For the purpose of health education, these theories can help us to understand how people learn, unlearn and relearn certain facts which are related to their habits, routines, behaviours, actions, decision-making and choices in the field of health and disease.

Learning can be defined as relatively permanent changes in behaviour potential occurring as the result of past experience (Lieberman,1974; Bandura,1969). It is important to note that learning affects the 'behaviour potential', and not necessarily the behaviour as such. There are many different types of learning processes.

Conditioning

This theory is built on natural, 'conditioned stimuli' occurring together with 'conditioned responses'. Translated into human learning situations, one could assume that some learning, especially in early childhood, takes the form of 'classical conditioning', as in the case of the use of the word 'bad' when it has been associated with certain actions, which will continue to affect a child even though circumstances change. It can also be assumed that a crucial element in learning is reinforcement by means of reward. This idea can be translated to human beings, who also learn by means of operant conditioning. With the introduction of technology for learning, the principle of reward is used to reinforce pupils in their learning process.

Social learning

From these first simple steps in understanding the process of learning in humans by analogies drawn from animal studies, further developments (Bandura et al.,1969) took into consideration the complexity of human responsiveness to different stimuli, at different times, in different situations and in performing different social roles. This has resulted in theories related to *social learning,* of which Bandura is one of the recognised exponents. Traditional theories depicted learning as a consequence of direct experience, whereas in real life people learn at least as much by observing and modeling on others, as from experiencing something themselves. Modeling, as a part of observational learning, includes attentional processes (identifying the behaviour that one wants to model), retention processes (observation will be effective if the observer commits it to memory), motor reproduction processes (reproducing the model's behaviour will depend on the existing skills of the observer), reinforcement and motivational processes (reproduction of learned behaviour from a model requires positive reinforcement, which will result in the observer's motivation to actually perform the desired behaviour).

Any attempt to translate this understanding into a practical learning situation will soon reveal that just providing a model copy is not enough to create similar behavioural patterns in others. On the other hand, a model person who repeatedly demonstrates desired responses, instructs others to reproduce them, physically prompts the behaviour when it fails to occur, and then administers powerful rewards, will eventually elicit corresponding responses in most observers. The crucial factor in this process is 'repeatedly', which may mean anything from a few to hundreds of demonstrations.

Reward is, however, only one of the many reinforcers which affects the outcome of a learning experience. Often, negative reinforcers are just as effective, such as punishment for the absence of particular behaviour. Reinforcement control plays an important part as a behaviour modification technique, based on the assumption that behaviour is controlled by its consequences, which may include direct experiences or symbolic social reinforcements. Some of the symbolic social reinforcements may include the approval of others, money, social success, etc.

Cognitive models

Not all human behaviour can be explained in terms of external stimulus and conditioned response consequences. Various cognitive factors play an important part in deciding what one observes, feels, and does in certain situations and at certain times. Cognition plays an important part in recognizing the links between stimuli and responses, and between responses and the consequences as reinforcements. Cognitive models of learning have therefore become increasingly influential, with the growth of attempts to improve learning ability through working on individuals' patterns of concepts and ideas. The recent increase of interest in computer-based artificial intelligence has also encouraged research into the ways in which people build up conceptual frameworks.

An aspect of cognitive control is the part that *belief* plays in the interpretation of experiences or observations. Very often the belief about a consequence overrides the actual experiences or observations of a consequence. One can, therefore, modify the statement that behaviour is controlled by its 'immediate' consequences, and replace this with 'anticipated' consequences. Belief and actuality do not always correspond, and this is an area in which learning can produce important results. Cognitive change through social learning is a dynamic process, based on a continuous interaction between behaviour and its controlling conditions. It is a two-way causal process between the environment and the individual, where one forms the other, and is in turn formed by the other.

Communication

In terms of health promotion and education, communication is interpreted as meaning an interaction between an individual and another individual, a group or a whole society. In this sense, it is a part of human behaviour and social interaction, and encompasses both verbal and non-verbal means of communication, and the relevant theories developed in these areas.

The simple approach of telling people what is best for them, in the hope that they will heed the advice, is recognised as being insufficient. The complexity of getting results is reflected in the analysis of the communication process as one of the central factors in health promotion and education.

In order to understand the different ways in which the concept of communications has been studied, it will be useful to mention some of the issues in research, which are relevant to planning health education and health promotion interventions:

- *The engineering model* – based on the development of communication technology; it consists of the sender +coding + the channel + decoding + the receiver. The engineering model was designed to answer such questions as: *"Who sends the message? Why has it been sent? How has it been sent? What has been sent to whom, and with what effect?"* The appeal of this model lay in its contribution to the rapidly growing interest in the effects and effectiveness of communication, using as its theoretical framework the widely accepted stimulus-response model of behaviour control and learning, and providing a basis for the development of a new scientific discipline of communication. It was influential even before the growth of new information and communication society.

- *Social orientation model* – is sensitive to problems of the social distance between the sender and the receiver; there may be a difference arising from their 'parochial' as compared with 'cosmopolitan' orientation to health care.

- *The role of 'noise'* - (general term for interference), or confusing issues, is very important in reducing the effectiveness of communication. The message sent may differ from the message received due to the effect of 'noise'.

- *The role of redundancy* - a counteracting factor to the negative effects of noise is that of 'redundancy', or the repetition of the message or its parts.

- *The two-step flow model* - is based on the concept of 'opinion leaders'; it states that the flow of information is through a medium (radio) to the opinion leaders and from them to the less active sections of the population. Subsequently, the concept of opinion leaders has changed into that of 'gate keepers', or people who hold the key positions in a communication network, and are influential in forming the social norms of that community.

- *Other models* - more recent studies have concentrated on *language* as one of the prerequisites for successful communication (syntactics, semantics and pragmatics); studies concerned with language acquisition have drawn attention to the possibility of the existence of a restricted period in human development during early childhood, which is optimal for language acquisition, with consequential difficulties in learning in later life if the opportunities are missed; other studies have highlighted the differentiation in the type of communication code (elaborated or restricted) learned during socialization, according to the social class and school environment of the receiver; attempts have been made to establish the existence of a universal 'language acquisition device' (LAD) inherent in every human being, which would account for the underlying similarities of different languages, and would also explain how a child acquires language skills so quickly; the advent of computers suggested new models, such as the cybernetic model, which is characterized by its feed-back mechanism.

Decision-making theories

The decision-making process is activated in situations where there are no dominant norms (normative behaviour) and a person is faced with a number of choices or alternatives (McGrew & Wilson, 1982). It is currently accepted that decision-making processes depend not only on the method of transmitting information, but to a large extent on the contents of the message. For this reason, health education messages need to be carefully adjusted to the perceived needs of the receivers, so as to maximize the probability of their making the desired choice. The advantages of recommending actions have in the past been over-stressed, as well as its failures when the recommended solution is rejected. One way of enhancing the recommended solution has been by using fear. A number of studies have examined the effects of using fear as an instrument for frightening people into desired actions. It was soon realised that there is no such thing as 'optimal' fear and that people are either frightened or not. Fear tends to act as an inhibitor and the process of rationalization occurs, with no action taking place. The validation of the experience by others has been found to play an important part, and the role of an immediate social network, as well as the professions, has been found of greatest importance. Since any decision may be followed by a feeling of regret or uncertainty, it has been found that any message transmitted by the mass media needed a follow-up reinforcement to counteract the effects of such cognitive dissonance, which is a result of the conflict between attitudes and actions, and which can be resolved in many different ways.

In more general terms, decision-making has been of interest to many professions and to different branches of science. Two main types of models used in the understanding of decision-making: *static* and *dynamic* models can be distinguished.

Static models have been based on the postulate that individuals will attempt to maximise the utility of a decision (*subjective expected utility* or SEU). Another model of great importance has been the deterministic *transitive model,* which postulates that if a person prefers A to B, and prefers B to C, then he/she will automatically prefer A to C. These models have not been sufficiently universal in explaining every combination of a decision-making process, and have been gradually replaced by *stochastic* models, where a person acts as though they are calculating the probability for each stage of the process.

Dynamic models consider decision-making as a function of the interaction of environmental and personal factors, where the environment may be stable and the information changes, or the environment changes and the information is stable.

The basis of most personal decision-making models is the assumption that the process can be only studied if an ideal situation is used as the base-line, and the divergences evident in the actual process are then examined. The base-line assumption has often been that a person is represented by 'economic man', who is characterised by total rationality, and controls total information about the subject related to making a decision. In practice, this would mean that this ideal person would be rational in the sense that he/she would try to maximise the benefits and minimise the cost involved in a decision, and that the information he/she has would, in every case, influence the decision within this framework. The studies of deviation from this ideal state have, therefore, concentrated on the emotional or other influences which affect this total rationality, or the amount and quality of information that has coloured the decision in question. Since the available information is concerned with alternatives on offer, the studies have also included the assessment processes in the light of preferences and constraints.

There are many ways a decision-maker, for example, a smoker, can obtain information about a health matter. For instance, a smoker may learn about the harmful effects of smoking cigarettes from a friend, from his/her doctor, by reading about it in the paper, by attending a lecture or in a number of other ways. The common factor in this is that a smoker receives information, and is faced with the decision of whether to act or not. Therefore, the decision-making process will form the core of the system within which an individual operates with regard to risk, illness and health.

In order to facilitate the understanding of the decision-making process, a simple diagram shows the pre-decision and the post-decision aspects of the decision-making process based on receiving information, making a decision and undertaking an action:

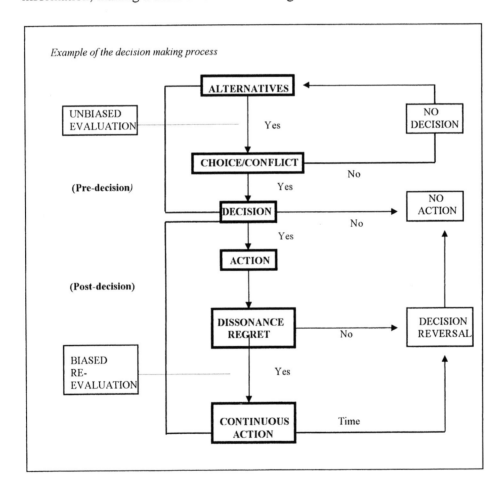

Pre-decision process - We start with the assumption that a person is faced with several mutually exclusive alternatives; because each has a certain attractiveness, a state of conflict exists. It is necessary to make a choice between two possible decisions: if the conflict is not resolved, no action will follow and the person will continue to assess different alternatives which are facing him or her; if the conflict is resolved, then the action will take place. The more similar the attractiveness of choices, the greater will be the conflict. In resolving it, the decision-maker will carry out an evaluation of each alternative, which one can assume is an objective or unbiased process. It will result in collecting additional information and building of divergence between the alternatives in order to make the choice easier.

Post-decision process - The decision made is equivalent to a commitment, based on the alternative chosen. If the decision is negative, then there will be no action, and the person will continue to evaluate various alternatives, or just abandon the whole idea. If, however, the positive decision is followed by an action, then the person has entered a state characterised by the existence of cognitive dissonance. The concept of cognitive dissonance postulates that every individual strives towards consistency within himself, both of opinions and behaviour. When inconsistency or dissonance exists, being psychologically uncomfortable, it will motivate the person to try to reduce it and achieve consonance. It can be reduced by changing one of the two elements between which dissonance exists, by changing the environmental influence or by changing the opinion through additional information. The process of reduction is considered to be biased and subjective: a person will try to reduce the dissonance by re-evaluating the alternatives and their attractiveness; the person may not be able to reduce it and then may reverse the decision, or, if that is not practical, may continue to have a feeling of regret about the choice that was made.

Behaviour in uncertainty

Many diseases have been found to be related to human behaviour, or dependent on a human action. A certain pattern of diet can result in under-nourishment or even overt disease; the early recognition of a lump in the breast, considered as a serious symptom, may result in the timely seeking out of medical advice and a considerable improvement in the eventual outcome. In the former case we talk about behaviour, and in the latter about an action, which may be defined as behaviour that is not merely a response but has a specific meaning or intention. The behaviour-action continuum illustrates a set of processes and influences derived from institutionalised or new knowledge about illness and health threats. Institutionalised knowledge is reflected in social expectations or norms about the preservation of health and the prevention and cure of illness. These norms are internalised by individuals as routines or habits, and become a part of the role performance that accompanies a specific social position or status.

New knowledge reaches the individual, either as a part of new or modified norms, or as a set of new alternatives, which may form the basis for a decision about the preservation of health, and the prevention or cure of a disease. The setting in which an individual is located is a powerful influence of the type of knowledge involved. New insights arising from medical discoveries about health threats may take time to become integrated into institutionalised knowledge and formalized norms. The reason for this is that not all the new discoveries are the result of aetiological studies (studies of causation). There are many cases where the new insight is the result of epidemiological studies (studies of the distribution of a problem in a population). Whereas in the former case it is possible to assert a causal relationship, in the latter case it is possible to establish only a statistical probability of the association between an individual manifesting a trait or behaviour and a risk or a disease. When this is the case, the individual is forced to assess the evidence when deciding whether or not to undertake a specific action, and without any threat of sanctions or other forms of social coercion. Health education has so far been mainly engaged in transmitting information to people about new discoveries related to the prevention of diseases, together with the recommended measures for the reduction of the attached risk. So far, the 'message transmission' approach has had relatively little success, in spite of the obvious logic of the arguments used.

The main problem in making a choice based on epidemiological studies or population probabilities is the theoretical inability to translate population probability to individual probability. New insight into this problem has been gained by studies of decision-making and of choice between several existing alternatives. Cohen (1972) made an early and important contribution to the understanding of these problems. He provided an insight into the assessment of the subjective or 'psychological' probability attached to statistical evidence about a health threat, as perceived by an individual when confronted with a health education message recommending a behavioural change. He also contributed to the understanding of problems related to receiving, understanding and acting upon a message received by the introduction of the concept of thresholds: the information threshold, the psychological probability threshold and the action threshold.

The information threshold - The first question to be faced is the type and quantity of information a person must receive before even starting to relate it to himself, and starting to assess the utility of the recommended change, against the disutility of the discomfort accompanying such a step.

It is a well-known fact that knowledge as such is not in most cases sufficient to initiate the desired action. Following the interpretations given by Cohen (1972). It would appear that various people need different amounts of information before they reach their information threshold. Some may, however, make their decision 'instantaneously'. In other cases more information may be needed, or information with certain 'weight', before the threshold is reached.

Psychological probability threshold - Once the information threshold has been passed, a person will start to assess the possibility and the probability of a threat affecting him, and what the consequences might be. Cohen (1964) drew a clear distinction between the objective or mathematical probability of an event occurring, and the subjective or psychological probability a person attaches to that event. This problem has been largely neglected in health educational studies, and Cohen's work in this area represents a major contribution to health education.

One of the clues to the way people assess information about a probable risk to their health can be derived from the description Cohen gives of a person's translation of a population probability to his own personal (or sample) probability. According to probability theory, this cannot be done, since by definition a population probability can never be attributed to any specific event or individual in that population. There is the empirical evidence that in spite of the inability to translate population probability into individual probability, people daily try to guess what their chances are, when deciding upon an action.

How do people make such interpretations, and could the understanding of this process help health education? Cohen gives a very plausible explanation of this problem. The interpretation is not solely dependent on information about the population, but is also governed by people's ideas about the population (macrocosm), which they then translate to apply to themselves (microcosm). These ideas can be coloured by different influences such as ethical and aesthetic beliefs, as well as by one's own image. People can overestimate the probability of something that is considered to be beautiful or good, or can be over-optimistic. The translation of a person's image about the macrocosm into events concerning the microcosm has also been described by Suchman (1965), although in a different context. He related people's behaviour to their orientation: 'parochial' and 'cosmopolitan'. People with a parochial orientation showed a low level of medical knowledge; their knowledge was based on popular beliefs and personal experiences, and was acquired through informal sources; in illness they showed a high level of dependence on their immediate social environment (family and friends); they also showed a high level of scepticism about the medical care system and its agents. The cosmopolitans showed a high level of medical knowledge based on scientific evidence, acquired through formal sources such as the educational system or scientific literature; in illness they showed a low level of dependence on family and friends, and they were not at all sceptical about the health care system or their agents. When health education information is transmitted through public channels and its arguments are based on scientific concepts such as probability, the cosmopolitans are more likely to accept it than the parochials. This has been supported by studies of the utilisation of health services, and the modification of behaviour.

Lack of willingness to accept the arguments presented by health educators in favour of a change in behaviour may also be due to the misinterpretations of the probabilistic statements made. People in general have difficulties in differentiating between the 'possibility' and the 'probability' of an event occurring. This may be because it is usual for people to reason that something may or may not happen, i.e. that they will become ill or will stay well. This 'either-or' approach is treated as a 50 : 50 probability. The fallacy, however, is that these two events need not be equiprobable. The realistic interpretation would be, that although they can or cannot become ill, if they smoke their chance of becoming ill is twenty times higher than for non-smokers.

Another common fallacy is to treat discrete events as a sequence of events instead of teaching each one separately. When told that smoking in pregnancy may harm the foetus (Baric and MacArthur, 1977), women who had smoked during their previous pregnancy and had a healthy baby, in general disregarded such information. They believed that since it did not happen before, it 'cannot' happen now. On the other hand, it is known that parents with one Downs syndrome baby find it very difficult to believe that the next baby will not also be affected.

A relevant story was reported in *The Times* (23.9.1977), about an air crash in which the aircraft was split in two and half of the passengers were killed. A survivor from Turkey, in describing the accident concluded "Having survived the accident, I think I am now 'insured' against tragic happenings like this and won't be fatally involved in other aircraft crashes. I travel a lot by air". In Cohen's terms, the person must have obviously been an optimist, since if he had been a pessimist he could have equally logically reasoned, that since he had survived one crash, in the next one he would most certainly be killed.

The action threshold - Whether or not a person will undertake an action, after passing through the information and psychological probability thresholds, will also depend on passing through the action threshold. Even then it is still not certain what kind of action will follow.

The first question, therefore, will be what makes a person undertake an action? Becker (1974), in a review, lists a number of models applied by various researchers in an attempt to find this answer. A popular, and probably most widely used model in health education, was the Health Belief Model described by Rosenstock (1974). It postulated that a health action depends on people's belief in their own susceptibility to the health threat; that the occurrence of disease would at least have an effect of moderate severity on some component of their lives; that taking some action would in fact be beneficial, by reducing their susceptibility to the condition, or if the disease did occur, by reducing its severity; and that it would not entail overcoming important psychological barriers such as cost, pain, convenience and embarrassment. This model has been used in a number of retrospective, prospective and intervention studies, but was found to have descriptive rather than predictive value. Later an additional factor was included, i.e. the 'cue', which seems to be most important in triggering off an action, even if all the other factors are present. There have been several criticisms of this model: it does not include motivation as a factor; each person will provide his/her own cue if he/she decides to act; the factors in the model have not been standardised; they do not represent discrete units, etc. Becker also discusses other models related to this problem, some of which employ the notion of behaviour in uncertainty and psychological probability, related to making a choice. It seems, however, that the complete understanding of the psychological mechanisms which prompt a person to undertake an action still eludes us, and that each of the models mentioned explains only a part of the process without providing a complete answer.

Once a decision has been made and an action follows, we are faced with the problem of what kind of action it will be. An intervention study carried out among pregnant women (Baric, MacArthur and Sherwood, 1976), with the aim of policy information about the dangers of smoking during pregnancy, illustrates this point. A doctor in an ante-natal clinic talked with a number of pregnant women about the dangers to their unborn child, in an attempt to persuade them to give up smoking during pregnancy. In an interview in their homes, eleven weeks after the intervention, it was found that 52% of the women had reacted and did undertake some action. Although they each received the same kind of information, supported by similar kinds of arguments, the range of their reactions was considerable: 10% stopped smoking, 7% stopped but started again, 24% reduced and 11% increased the number of cigarettes smoked. The rest (48%) reported no change.

From all the studies cited, as well as from other literature, it seems obvious that the problem of making a decision that will result in a recommended action is much more complex than would appear from the existing models currently in use. It has also been shown that there is no such thing as a 'health action' or 'health behaviour', but that we are dealing with specific reactions of individuals to specific health threats or disease symptoms. One person may make up his mind 'instantaneously' when confronted with the facts, whereas another may need a long time and a vast amount of information before even considering the possibility of acting. One individual may react negatively to too little information about one health threat, and also negatively to too much information about another threat. It is also known that a low level of perceived susceptibility may inhibit one kind of action (vaccination), whereas too high a level of perceived susceptibility may inhibit or delay some other action (breast examination).

Within a setting, characterised by a power structure there are many actors who are directly or indirectly involved in decision-making relevant to health issues. These decisions may be about their own health or the health of others in the setting. They may be a part of the policy and strategy within this setting or a part of the interaction between individuals. Knowing the background to the decision-making process should enable better adjustment of interventions to the needs of the setting and the individuals within that setting.

Socialization

The birth of a child can be considered from two different points of view: from the point of view of the society or social organization into which the child has been born and from the point of view of the child itself. For society, it implies providing ways and means of integrating the child into the existing social system, with the fewest possible disruptions and threats to the system; whereas for the child it implies activating all the inherited biological and psychological attributes, for the purpose of understanding the surrounding world and adjusting to its demands, as well as learning how to survive in it.

Although there is no generally accepted single definition of *society*, for our purpose it will suffice to describe it as an "aggregate of human beings of both sexes and all ages bound together into a self-perpetuating group and possessing its own more or less distinctive institutions and culture...." (Gould & Kolb, 1964, p.674). *Culture* consists of patterns of behaviour, constituting the distinctive achievements of human groups, including their embodiments and artifacts, as well as ideas and their attached values. *Values* denote the shared cultural standards, according to which the objects of attitudes, desires and needs can be compared and judged.

Institutions

Because society is a self-perpetuating system, ways and means have evolved to ensure continuity. The social environment, with its comparative stable continuity, is man-made and not based on any biological determinants. Due to the instability of the human organism, it becomes imperative to provide a stable social environment with a well-defined *social order*, which is again, the product of human activities, and not based on any 'natural laws'.

In order to explain the 'social order' into which people are born, and which they consider to exist outside themselves as an *objective reality*, in spite of the fact that it has been humanly created in the first place, it is useful to trace the way an activity becomes institutionalised.

When a human activity is repeated frequently and produces the desired results with a minimum of effort, it becomes *habitualised*. Although a person has drives, which if not satisfied create tensions, he or she must learn a socially acceptable way of satisfying them, and thus relieving such tensions. Habitualisation provides the direction and specialization of activity, which can reduce the accumulated tensions that result from *undirected drives*. By accepting habitualised behaviour, the need for *decisions* is reduced because of pre-set patterns of behaviour for certain standard situations. Habitualisation also implies that the same pattern of behaviour can be applied in any future situation. By reducing tensions and the need for decisions, Habitualisation supports the stability of the external world, frees people for experimentation with innovative solutions, and creates the basis for the *predictability* of human behaviour. When habitualised behaviour becomes a part of a social interaction, and when there is reciprocal typification of habitualised behaviour between several actors engaged in a social interaction, then such habitualised behaviour becomes *institutionalized*.

Institutionalised behaviour in a society deals with some basic problems of that society, and, in this sense represents the institutions of that society. Some of the most common areas of institutionalised behaviour in any society include language, work, gender and territoriality. Institutions involve the regulation of an individual's behaviour according to some definite pattern, including a normative ordering and regulation, upheld by sanctions which support these norms.

Thus, by definition, institutions exercise *control* over human conduct by setting predetermined patterns of behaviour. Control raises the problem of an individual's compliance or deviance from the existing norms. The mechanism of sanctions in the case of *deviance* is generally described as the system of *social control.*

Functions of socialization

Ongoing social systems integrate new members so that they fit into the existing structure without disruption. Socialization thus represents an important instrument of social control, by means of which societies ensure that the newly integrated individuals conform to social norms inherent in the institutions of the relevant society.

A socialized individual internalizes the 'right' meaning attached to the relevant behavioural patterns. *Legitimization* refers to all devices that maintain the taken-for-granted reality of the society counteracting any potential questioning. This implies that the fundamental structures of a society within which social experience takes place are not questioned but are accepted as seemingly natural and self-evident conditions of everyday life. One of the main characteristics of institutions is their *historicity.* Institutions exist before a person is born, and will be there long after he or she dies. They are handed on in terms of a tradition, without the person's awareness of how and why they were evolved.

Institutions evolve through the interaction of individuals and become the *objective reality* for every new member born into that society, confronting him or her as an external and coercive fact. Such a world becomes a 'social world' in terms of comprehension and firmness it achieves in a person's consciousness. For a child it becomes the 'real' world, and is not easily changed by individual efforts. By internalizing such an objective reality, the child develops his/her *subjective reality*, which represents his personal interpretation of the world around him.

The adjustment between the objective and subjective realities is central to the process of socialization. Because the objective reality of the outside world undergoes constant changes, and because human biological development continues after birth and represents a long-term process, every viable society must develop procedures for reality-maintenance to maintain the symmetry between the objective and the subjective reality.

Because of the incorporation of new experience, new knowledge and new interpretations of existing knowledge, the maintenance of objective reality is constantly being threatened. Since the individual may not always be successful in adjusting the balance between the objective and subjective reality, more reliable procedures for routine and crisis-management exist.

In the small-scale social systems of pre-industrial societies, the objective reality internalised during early childhood did not change much. As the child grew up, the skills and knowledge acquired during childhood largely sufficed for its future roles in that society. In the complex systems of industrialized societies, the period of acquisition of special skills and knowledge extends into adulthood. Because of this we can differentiate two qualitatively diverse aspects of socialization: primary and secondary or formal socialization.

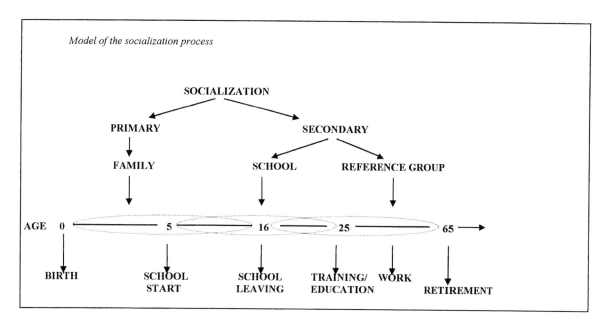

Primary socialization takes place within the family into which a child is born, lasts from birth through early childhood, and includes socially defined learning sequences, based on biological growth, and differentiated according to gender and the various social characteristics of the family. Through primary socialization, the child internalizes the values and norms mediated through significant others, who in this case are parents or parent substitutes. For the child, there is no choice of significant others or of the social world it enters, and at first the family represents the totality of 'the world'. The main characteristic of primary socialization is the child's identification with significant others, with whom it develops a very strong affective relationship. This is the period when attitudes are formed. The values, norms, routines, attitudes and habits internalised during that period, because of their affective aspect, are of a lasting nature, and can be changed in later years only with great difficulty and by means of special processes.

Secondary or formal socialization takes place during the later parts of childhood and adolescence, as well as early adulthood. Because of the division of labour and differentiation of social roles, there is a need for the social distribution of skills and knowledge in a society. In this way an individual acquires role-specific skills and knowledge and specific languages, and is able to take his or her place in that society. The main characteristic of the secondary socialization process is the lack of emotional involvement (with certain exceptions) with the agent of socialization who usually has a socially recognized and formally legitimized role in that society. The process is characterized by formality and anonymity, and often includes a ritual aimed at legitimizing the new status acquired by the individual. A good example is the child's education, carried out in formally recognized schools, by teachers, transmitting special skills and knowledge for the fulfillment of future roles, and including examinations and formal ceremonies of graduation on completion of the process.

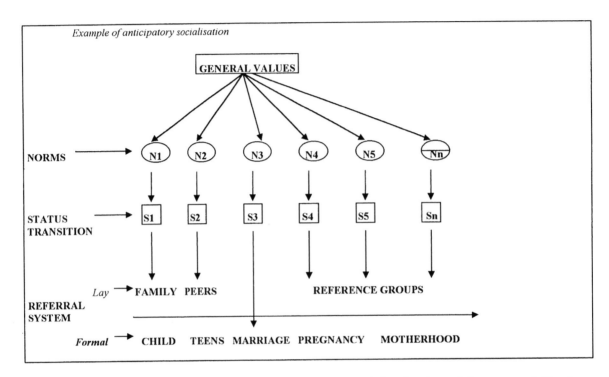

Sometimes an important aspect of secondary or formal socialization is anticipatory socialization, which can also be described as the positive orientation of individuals to non-membership groups. Individuals, who adopt the values of a group to which they do not belong, but to which they aspire, are considered to be undergoing *anticipatory socialization*. The system may make provisions for anticipatory socialization, as in the case of medical students. They spend some time during their formal education in hospitals, stay with general practitioners and learn, generally speaking, how to act and behave like the doctors with whom they identify. In this case, anticipatory socialization is considered to be functional, but in a closed group, where the individual cannot gain acceptance as a member, and loses his place in the old group, it would be dysfunctional. This is the case of the marginal person who does not fully belong to any specific group. From the standpoint of the group, which the person is aiming to leave, anticipatory socialization can be dysfunctional, whereas from the point of view of the society, it is functional, because it reinforces the structure, and provides a positive orientation for certain out-group norms. An example of anticipatory socialization is preparation for motherhood in pregnancy.

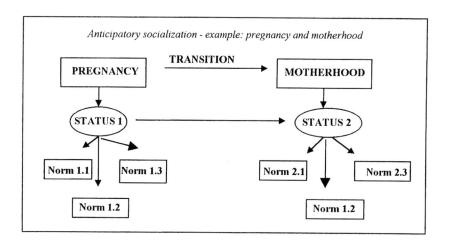

Anticipatory socialization - example: pregnancy and motherhood

Counselling

A definition of behavioural counselling is: *"a process of helping people to learn how to solve certain interpersonal, emotional and decision problems"* (Krumboltz & Thorsen,1976). A key idea in the definition is to 'learn', which emphasizes that counselling is about helping the clients to acquire certain skills or levels of competence in dealing with their problems.

The phrase 'behavioural counselling' indicates that the result of counselling is a change in behaviour. Another key phrase in the definition is 'how to solve', which implies that the aim of counselling is to enable clients to become independent and self-reliant problem solvers. The clients' independence will be ultimately manifested in their ability to give up their dependence on the counsellor. In this way, clients can become more self-reliant and independent, and better able to solve their own problems. The other key words are 'certain....problems', which make it clear that the clients must be able to diagnose problems and learn to accept that not all problems can be solved, or solved by the clients alone.

Counsellors can help clients in a number of problem areas, such as improving their interpersonal relationships, solving some emotional problems, learning about problem solving and decision making. Clients can learn to change some habits such as smoking and overeating, and learn to take better care of their bodies. They can also learn how to overcome shyness, stress and depression, sexual dysfunction, alcoholism, compulsive gambling and drug abuse, as well as fears and anxieties. Because of the great variety of the problems, counsellors must specialize, and thus will become experts in a specific field of problems presented by clients.

Counsellors can be involved in helping people to solve existing problems, or they can help people to prevent certain problems before they occur. They learn from their remedial work about the variety of problems that could have been avoided, and can become involved in preventive counselling.

The main aim of counselling is twofold. On the one hand, the client should learn to make decisions wisely and to be able to change his/her own behaviour to produce the desired consequences, in order to assume control of his/her own life. The question arises as to why so many people do not have these skills and need help. The main reason is that these skills are a part of the socialization process, and have to be learned. The environment in which some people have grown up does not provide opportunities for learning such skills. For example, some environments do not provide individuals with sufficient rewards for certain kinds of behaviour. Without such reinforcement, it is doubtful whether a person will learn how to take control of his/her own life, or how to avoid feelings of powerlessness, depression and alienation.

On the other hand, in certain groups or environments, some forms of negative behaviour are accepted and reinforced. The consequence is that a person conforms in the group but is 'deviant' as far as the rest of the society is concerned. The person may not realize that there is a problem at all. In some environments, excessive punishment may be used as a form of social control, which can leave people with phobias or some form of deviant behaviour. The result may be an exaggeration of their problems, which then become increasingly difficult to solve. Some people may not have had the opportunity to learn to recognize the signals or cues that indicate whether certain behaviour is appropriate or not. Without the sensitivity to reading and reacting to social cues, a person may continue with a pattern of behaviour, without realizing that there is any need to change it.

In general terms one can define three main areas where counselling is being widely employed: decision-making; in altering maladaptive behaviour (behavioural deficit or excess, inappropriate behaviour, fears and anxieties and physical problems), and prevention.

One of the most crucial skills that a counselor needs is an ability to help the client develop decision-making skills. For these skills an eight-step model is appropriate:

- Formulate the problem by specifying the client's goals and values;
- Commit time and effort;
- Generate alternative solutions;
- Collect information about the alternatives;
- Examine the consequences of the alternatives;
- Re-evaluate goals, alternatives and consequences;
- Eliminate the least desirable alternatives until a tentative choice is made;
- Generalize the decision-making process to apply to new problems.

Counsellors have at their disposal a great number of techniques (it has been estimated over 30), which range from information-giving and relaxation methods, to counter-conditioning and token exchange systems.

Some recent developments in counselling methods include: treating fears through conditioning experience as well as imagination; managing fears rather than avoiding them; using coping models rather than mastery models; encouraging self-control rather than external control; using covert and cognitive behaviour as well as overt, observable behaviour; employing prevention as well as remedial methods, etc. One of the main difficulties encountered in counselling is the formulation of goals from the problems presented, which may take the following forms: the problem is someone else's behaviour, the problem is expressed as a feeling, the problem is the absence of a goal, the problem is that the desired behaviour is undesirable, the problem is that the client does not know his or her behaviour is inappropriate, the problem is a choice conflict, or the problem is a vested interest in not identifying any problems.

In some situations, people have helped others just by talking to them, and listening to their problems. Once this activity became formalized, the profession of counsellors was born. Since then a number of developments have occurred, and counselling activities have been shared among a number of professions such as social workers, doctors, nurses, dietitians, and others.

The main characteristics which counsellors all need include empathy, acceptance and genuineness. They need to conduct themselves professionally and take responsibility for the consequences of their work by keeping in touch with the clients until the solution of the problem has been achieved. Since counselling became recognized as a professional activity, people engaged in it have needed special training. Numerous professions find themselves in the situation of being involved in counselling, and various courses offering them the necessary skills. There are other areas of commerce or industry where counselling has been used as a part of looking after the health of their workers. In addition, preventive counselling has been introduced by industry as a service to employees who are facing redundancies and job loss. It was found that losing a job is less stressful if the person in question can become adjusted to this fact with the help of a counsellor.

The starting point in the counselling interaction is when a client presents his/her 'problem', which can be an undesirable habit, a crisis, an anxiety, a frustration, or any other kind of concern. This, however, is not necessarily a problem which has an accompanying solution. It is more of a problem situation, which can either be changed, or needs to be coped with. This situation is often due to missed opportunities or to the unused potential of the client. In other cases, where there is no possibility of solving the problem, the helper will assist the client to handle the situation better. In practice one can differentiate among stages through which the helping process must pass in the process of finding a solution (Egan, 1986).

Stage I is concerned with the identification of the problem by the client. It consists of: a) telling the story; b) screening, focusing and clarifying the problem, a process carried out by the client with the help of the helper; c) developing new perspectives on the problem.

Stage II is concerned with setting new goals, based on the new action-oriented understanding of the problem, the selection of one goal, as the result of the previous process of screening and focusing, and the development of a preferred scenario for action. This consists of a) the choice of a new scenario; b) critical assessment of that scenario; c) choice and commitment to specific actions.

Stage III is concerned with the development and implementation of strategies for reaching the agreed-upon goals. It consists of: a) brainstorming possible strategies for the chosen action; b) formulating a plan for the implementation of these strategies; and c) the action or implementing the decisions and commitments made by the client.

This model is cumulative, since success in stage II will depend on success in stage I, and stage III will depend on the successful completion of stages I and II. In other words, the stages are integral parts of a dynamic process of interaction, which should be considered as a whole, and in which the stages are differentiated, for easier monitoring of the processes and the evaluation of outcomes.

It is important to bear in mind that the stages of the model presented should be treated as guidelines, along which an interaction could progress. They should not be applied rigidly, since this could destroy the spontaneity of the client's involvement in solving his/her problem. The counsellor must have skills which will enable him/her to show empathy and explore the problems in greater depth, to confront the client with different aspects of the problems, and to move the client towards undertaking the agreed upon action.

The training of counsellors in the application of this approach includes the understanding of the procedure, observation of a skilled counsellor who is applying it in a real life situation, step-by-step supervised practice, and extended practice in real life situations.

The implications for HP/HE

The health behaviour of an individual is a function of the socio-environmental and personal factors. In terms of socialization, the environmental factors include the social creation of an 'objective reality' into which a child is born and is being integrated. The personal factors include the integration of the objective reality in the form of the subjective reality of an individual. Knowledge, attitudes and skills related to health will form a part of the socialization process. This implies that the interventions on a personal level will have to take place during the various processes of socialization (primary, secondary, anticipatory, as well as resocialization) and that they will depend on the competence of the socializing agents (parents, teachers, doctors, etc.), in creating an objective reality, conducive to the maintenance of health and prevention and the management of diseases.

The personal methods of intervention thus include the learning ability of individuals, the interchange between the individuals based on their ability to communicate and the support provided by friends, important others and professionals in situations when the subjective reality does not match the objective reality, or needs to be modified for the purpose of maintenance of health, prevention and management of disease.

In a family setting h ealth promotion deals primarily with the creation of the appropriate objective reality, health education influences the integration of this objective reality into the subjective reality of an individual and will provide support for a conformist behaviour and actions.

Introduction

Most human activities take place in social groups. Since settings are always associated with social groups, the group approach is vitally important in working with settings. Health promotion and education can utilize group processes and mechanisms for the attainment of the set goals related to health improvement and disease prevention, management and treatment (Douglas, 1970,1976; Klein, 1963; Cartwright and Zander, 1953; Dean and Rosen, 1955; Thelan, 1954; Moore, 1987; Pfeiffer and Jones, yearly). There are different ways of classifying groups for the purpose of better understanding of their potential for health promotion and education. According to the type of group, one can differentiate between:

- *pre-existing groups* - such as families, school classes, professional groups etc.;

- *newly created groups* - such as learning groups, decision and action groups, self-help groups, therapeutic groups, etc.

There are several important characteristics to be taken into account when using a group method for the purpose of health promotion and education:

- *group cohesiveness* - which denotes the mutual attraction of its members, and the level of a member's identification with group values and goals;

- *group pressures* - which influence members' conformity to group values and norms, and lead to changes in attitudes and acceptance of group goals;

- *group goals* - which can be imposed or shared, and which will depend on members' commitment and actions;

- *group structure* - which will help in understanding the power structure within the group, the communication processes and the role of leadership within a group.

Since most social interactions take place in groups, the social and behavioural sciences have studied groups, resulting in the development of methodologies and a whole set of theoretical explanations concerning the structure, processes and outcomes of group interactions.

Large Groups

People very often find themselves as members of some large group or gathering which meets for various specific reasons. Some of the most common reasons are set out below:

Transmission of information

One aim of a large gathering or meeting can be to transmit information to a group of people about some issue, problem, event or topic of general interest. It usually takes the form of a meeting with a speaker, as in the case of political gatherings, or it can take the form of a lecture given by a speaker on a specific topic. The advantage of this kind of interaction is the possibility of reaching a large number of people in a limited space of time, using only one speaker.

Knowledge sharing

The sharing of knowledge throughout large groups is a very common occurrence. Most of the learning that takes place in schools is done in classes, which represent a large group situation. The methods of acquisition, as well as assessment, form the basis of our educational system.

Entertainment

Most entertainment that includes a live audience is performed in large groups. The processes involved are well known and tested by many entertainers, who can measure their success by immediate feedback from the audience.

Sometimes, a large group can have all the three elements simultaneously present: transmission of information, acquisition of knowledge and entertainment. This aspect is very important in evaluating large group performance, and has to be reflected in the definition of the aims of that group, to include all the three aspects. It could well happen that the success of a group aiming to transmit information is assessed on the basis of its entertainment value.

Summing up

Most large meetings do not produce decisions or commitments among participants, since they do not have a built-in mechanism for member participation, which is the basis for a decision making process. Voting (by ballot or show of hands) is the most common form of decision-making in a large gathering where that is appropriate. Informal large audiences rarely have built in mechanisms for interacting and receiving feedback from members. The chairman can be the expert, or can be accompanied by an expert who provides the contents of a lecture. The feedback is usually restricted to inviting members to 'ask questions' or 'give comments'. The response is limited to those who feel secure enough to stand up in a large meeting, or who feel that they know more than the expert knows and want to show it to others.

One way to enable members of a large meeting to provide feedback is a method of participation in which the chairman asks the audience to form groups of six or seven members sitting together, who turn to face each other and have between five and ten minutes to discuss the lecture and agree on the most important point they would like to make. The chairman then invites a representative of each group to present the point, or raise a question from the group. In this way, the chairman can ensure feedback from most of the audience, who will have a feeling of active participation in the meeting.

Another way to capitalize on the existing potential in an audience is to invite members with specific interests or expertise to form a sub-group or a sub-committee, and thus ensure the continuation of work on the issues raised at the meeting.

In the past, the use of large meetings was avoided by 'progressive' health education and gave way to work in small groups as the method of preference. The importance of mass meetings is now realized, although for different purposes. These meetings need to be seen as an important part of a selection of methods, especially for health promotion, and should be evaluated in that context.

Small Groups

A person living in a society cannot avoid being a member of a number of small groups, where the interaction between the members is most intense, and the group membership can be of a lasting duration. Because of the pervasiveness of small groups, small group research or the study of group dynamics has been one of the major interests in social sciences, as well as health education and health promotion. There are many publications reporting the findings of such research and dealing with group processes and mechanisms, as well as the behaviour of group leaders, group observers and group members (Baric, 1996, pp.275-289).

Family groups

Everybody is born into a family, and in most cases creates a family of their own in later life. The family group is a situation where primary socialization occurs and children learn how to survive in a social environment, and acquire values, knowledge and skills relevant for their immediate and future roles. Because of this, the competence of a family to raise a healthy new generation is very important, and has been the target for health promotion and health education for a long time.

Studies of family groups have developed a classificatory system, which differentiates types of families according to a number of dimensions: membership, cycle of family development, role relationship between members, social class, geographical location, culture, religion, income, education, etc. Most of those dimensions have been found to be associated with the health of the members of a family, and have been used by health promotion and health education in planning their interventions.

A special aspect of studying the family group relationships has been their interaction with the health care system and especially with their family practitioners. The existing literature related to the group aspects of this relationship has concentrated on social support and the diffusion effect of various experiences shared by family members. One should realize that family groups are linked to other groups through their kin and social networks. Their kin relationship can be defined as close-knit or loose-knit according to the intensity and proximity of kin members to a family unit. All these elements play an important part when planning a health promotion and education intervention based on a family unit instead of an individual. Different methods have been developed concentrating on raising family competence in dealing with health problems, and bringing up a healthy new generation.

Adolescent groups

A specific aspect of industrialized societies is the recognition of a special status given to adolescent groups, resulting in the development of the concept of an adolescent culture. A number of studies looking at peer groups have explored the relationships between the members of such groups in many areas of their social activities, such as material consumption, fashion, pop culture, sexual relationships, deviancy etc. Health studies concerned with this population group have been mainly concerned with the high mortality and morbidity rates in comparison with the general population and with the group's specific problems such as road accidents, smoking, drug abuse, teenage pregnancies, gang wars, crime, etc.

More recently a new form of health education and health promotion has been taking place in relation to this population group, resulting in the creation of a number of self-help groups dealing with health and social problems. The framework within which these problems occur may be home, school or work; each will have certain specific characteristics relevant to a health promotion and education intervention.

Adolescent groups reflect in a special and characteristic way the three important aspects of social structure: informal hierarchy, networks and systems (sociometric structures) and norms. There is no central task activity and no formal hierarchy of power or leadership. There can be leaders for specific activities, and the leadership role may rotate among the members according to their special talents or abilities.

Adolescent groups are of interest because of a number of special processes which are not evident in other types of groups: (a) there is no specific task, but joint activities are devised, which entail the kinds of interaction which meet the needs of members; (b) one of these needs is the establishing of an ego-identity, independent of the family of origin, which is reflected in the emphasis on clothes, the great self-consciousness and the concern about acceptance by members of the group; (c) sexual motivation is a major factor in adolescent groups, and is partly responsible for the intensity of attraction to the groups, and for their pairing structure; (d) there is, however, a common group task of acquiring together the social skills of dealing with the opposite sex, and dealing with adults.

All these characteristics are important when planning a health promotion or education intervention, which will have to consider very specific mechanisms and processes, as well as interests and motivation, characteristic for this population group.

Work-groups

In our society, most adults, especially males, are expected to work for their living, and high rates of unemployment create a category of people who cannot, or do not, meet these expectations. Even people at work are exposed to high levels of stress due to insecurity and the danger of losing their job. The part of the female population that works at home-making, has not a fully recognized legitimate and gainful occupation. This creates a different range of problems and stresses.

Health care at work is mainly concerned with the reduction of accidents and absenteeism from work. There are organization, using specific methods, which carry out health promotion and health education at work. There are various opportunities for workers to undergo health check-ups, and have their health regularly monitored, especially where they are exposed to some health hazards within the working environment. More recently, there have also been instances where the workers and employees have had access to counselling services because of the high levels of stress or conflict situations.

Unlike adolescent groups, the work group is primarily concerned with carrying out a task. To do this, the group has a formalized structure, with norms regulating the relationships between people occupying different statuses in a work-group. The assessment of the success or failure of a work-group is usually expressed in terms of levels of productivity quality or teamwork

The members of work-groups are characterized by having special knowledge or skills and have to undergo a process of training or education to be able to meet the expectations at work. This preparatory period is characterized by anticipatory socialization, where people learn what is expected of them in terms of performance and behaviour. This is when they learn about the norms governing relationships, as well as the ways of entering and leaving a working group. The social environment within which work-groups operate is usually clearly defined in terms of legal, economic and social norms. One of the problems arising from the social environment can be that a work-group, internally assessed as being highly successful, can disintegrate or be dissolved due to economic conditions in the environment.

It has been established that the most successful work-groups are those characterised by a high level of cohesion, which is reflected in high group morale. Some other groups, which are apathetic and erratic, show low cohesion and are also less successful in achieving the tasks. Some highly cohesive groups, such as strategic groups, related to union activities, are not necessarily positive with respect to production since their main task is to protect the rights of their members. More traditional groups may manifest high output and be moderately cohesive. They may have a cooperative attitude and can be highly productive. These characteristics apply to people in high status jobs who find it easier to perform joint tasks within an atmosphere of cooperation.

Studies of work-groups have looked at structure and power distribution by applying sociometric methods. They have looked at close relationships within sub-groups, the problems of identity with the group, or with the product and the security levels for members of the group. The leadership role acquires special meaning in terms of informal group structures as well as formal management structures.

Health promotion and education interventions have to take into account the complexity of group structures, the symbolic importance of group identity and the traumatic consequences of leaving a group. There have been some attempts at preventive counselling, not only in the case of planned redundancies but also for people leaving the group due to retirement. In some high-stress occupations this can have very dramatic consequences, for example, an exceptionally high death rate was noticed among airline pilots within the first five years of their retirement.

Committees, problem solving and creative groups

Most decisions in public life are reached as a result of committee work. The members are formally nominated, their tasks are regulated and the procedures are set out. The work is done by means of discussion, which is aimed at taking decisions and solving problems. Being a member of a committee adds prestige to an individual's standing in a society and that is one of the main motivational forces for constructive participation in the work of committees.

Interaction in committees is unlike interaction in most other groups. Although it is primarily verbal, non-verbal language plays a very important part, for example, when one has to catch the eye of the chairman to be allowed to speak. The interaction is highly regulated, with set rules applying to the language used in addressing the chair and other members, the duration and the frequency of speaking, as well as in terms of contents governed by the agenda.

Understanding the working of committees is very important, especially for health promotion, where one of the methods, i.e. lobbying, will depend on using this knowledge to attract attention and get a problem on the agenda of a committee. This method has so far been greatly neglected in health promotion and education training programmes, which have disregarded the fact that in some countries (e.g. USA, UK) there is a 'professional' group of lobbyists for hire, with a high level of skills in performing their job.

T-groups and therapy groups

The existence of these groups is due to the discovery by psychologists and psychiatrists that patients, when treated in groups, can show higher levels of recovery than when treated individually (Whittaker, 1965). There is a difference between T-groups and therapy groups, with the former being concerned with specialized training and the latter with the treatment of certain mental disorders. The processes and mechanisms involved in these groups are highly specialized and require a professionally qualified leader. The rules to be adopted are a part of the teaching and treatment methods developed by psychologists, educationalists and the medical profession.

Health promotion and education contents can be a part of the training programme of such groups, depending on the professional skills involved in training or health problems presented in the group. Health promotion and education related to mental health is increasingly becoming a specialisation in its own right, with practitioners requiring special qualifications.

Self-help groups

Trends in health promotion and education have come to place great emphasis on developing self-reliance among people and communities (Hatch and Kickbusch, 1983; Gartner and Riessmann, 1977). This trend reflects existing developments in the self-help movement in industrialized societies. We are witnessing a real explosion in the number of self-help groups, a phenomenon which has been attributed to the growth of technology, increased complexity of institutions, depersonalization of services, increased professionalisation of everyday life, and the alienation of individuals from society, their local community, their families, other people and even from themselves.

Self-help groups have made a significant contribution dealing with problems, which could not be or were not solved by other institutions. They provide a mechanism whereby individuals in a group setting can assume responsibility for their own bodies, psyches and behaviour, gain back a feeling of competence and self-respect, and help others to participate in the solving of shared problems.

There is a self-help group for nearly every major disease listed by the World Health Organization. The self-help health groups include: addictions, blood disorders, endocrine conditions, health maintenance groups, intelligence problems, infant mortality, mental illness, neuromuscular disorders, obesity, physical disabilities, sensory disorders, skin disorders, surgery, and many others. Some of the self-help groups have developed into whole movements, such as environmentalist groups, energy conservation groups, community groups, not to mention the whole range of consumer protection and political groups. Their numbers have grown to enormous proportions and, according to a rough estimate, there may be hundreds of thousands of self-help and mutual aid groups in the world. They range from Alcoholics Anonymous (membership over 750,000) to groups for parents who abuse their children, groups for older citizens, for parents of twins, for cancer patients, for people on diets, for drug abusers, parent education groups, Gamblers Anonymous, Overeaters Anonymous, etc. From HP/HE, it is useful to define the main characteristics of self-help groups as distinct from other groupings:

- they mostly originate spontaneously and are not imposed from outside;
- they involve person-to-person interaction and the active participation of the members;
- the decisions for actions are based on agreement among the members;
- the groups usually start from a feeling of powerlessness, and fulfil a need of the members jointly to solve some problems that they could not solve alone;
- the group in this way fulfils the need for a reference group, identification with other members with a common cause, and as a means of ego reinforcement.

Sometime self-help groups operate within a defined ideological framework, for example, women's groups, gay groups or some minority groups, etc. This variety is reflected in the many definitions of self-help groups, such as: a social movement; a spiritual movement or a secular religion; a phenomenon of the service society; an alternative care-giving system; a supplementary community; an agency of social control and resocialization; an organization of deviants and the stigmatised; a vehicle for coping with life transitions; a therapeutic method, etc.

A simpler classificatory system differentiates between groups that focus on self-improvement (e.g. Alcoholic Anonymous), and those that focus on changing social norms (e.g. gay liberation groups). This reflects the distinction between the group's view of: whether the problem lies with the individual or the social system.

Another way of differentiating among self-help groups is based on whether the aim is social improvement, or self-fulfilment and personal growth, including groups that undertake the role of advocacy, groups that aim to create alternative patterns of living, or groups that represent 'outcast havens' or refuges for desperate people who are trying to achieve protection from the pressures of life and society.

The implicit assumption in the self-help group movement is that it is composed of lay people (in the context of group aims), and the main question is what, if any, is the role of professionals in the working of such groups. This problem is highlighted in health promotion and education, where an accepted method is for health educators to initiate the creation of 'self-help' groups, for the solution of a number of health problems. Their role in this area has not been defined, nor empirically tested, so that at present there is a variety of ways in which health education professionals can operate within this movement. In some cases, such as with community workers, there is a conflicting trend for them to reject dependence on the formal system (although paid by that system), and to identify with the community groups and their members. This raises a key question: will the professionals attempt to dominate and socialize the self-help group into existing professional norms, or will the self-help group be independent, although co-operating with the professional structure? The danger is that a successful self-help movement may provide the authorities with the justification for cutting down services and reallocating resources, for example in the attempt to return the elderly and mental patients 'into the community'. Another danger is that members of a self-help group, in seeking independence from the system, may become overdependent on the group, which means that they have only replaced one type of dependency for another.

Any systematic research (observation or experimentation) concerning the self-help movement might contaminate its spontaneity, and affect processes in such a way that the findings would not be valid. Therefore, most insight into group work has been gained from anecdotal sources in a descriptive form. There are, however, some generalizations that can be made about the group processes involved:

Helper-therapy principle - in helping others one helps oneself most; in other words, within an Alcoholic Anonymous group, when one alcoholic helps another, he or she will help himself most to avoid the temptation of taking a drink; this is a basic principle in certain types of self-help groups where the 'reformee' must also perform the role of the 'reformer', and may gain most by playing this supportive and helping role. Thus, the most effective way for ex-smokers to avoid starting to smoke again is to take over an active role in helping others to stop smoking thus reinforcing their own non-smoking behaviour.

Learning by teaching - it is a well known fact that one learns most if one is committed to teaching others. This is true for academics as much as for children who are recruited to teach other children hygiene habits.

The group process - the success of any self-help group will to a large extent depend on the processes that are being activated within the group. A successful group will provide peer support and identification with other members; will give aims, objectives, limits and norms; will provide feedback and reinforcement; will help to integrate individuals and will help individuals to combat stigma and change their perception of self.

Consumer as producer - the role of consumers in the field of human services has been recognized, and it is well known that the productivity of the producers will depend on their interaction with consumers. This is because much that is essential in the human services (health care, education, etc.) depends on the involvement of the consumers. To be successful in learning, the pupil must be fully involved in the learning process; to be healthy, a person must be fully involved in preventing and managing illness and maintaining health. This consumer involvement is one of the main characteristics of self-help groups.

Behaviour Modification Clinics

One of the areas where health promotion and health education is becoming increasingly active is in dealing with problems that can only be solved by creating a special environment for the clients. As a result of this, a number of specialized behaviour modification 'clinics' have been established, dealing with such problems as dieting and weight loss, giving up smoking, increasing exercise, changing lifestyles, managing stress, etc.

Behaviour modification methods

It would be wrong to limit diagnosis of a behavioural problem to the efforts of the internal response-producing agents; a more appropriate approach examines interrelated control systems in which behaviour is determined by external stimulus events, by internal information-processing systems and regulatory codes, and by reinforcing response feed-back processes (Bandura, 1969).

This holistic approach allows for the complex definition of the problem, and requires a treatment regime, that may include several methods. This does not imply that the treatment disregards some of the conventional methods of behaviour modification, such as higher level conditioning and various aspects of social learning. It does, however, mean that the range of available methods has been considerably increased and allows for better results.

The first step in contemplating behaviour modification treatment is to define the aims and objectives in terms of the expected result. Since the concepts involved are theoretical constructs, they will also need to be defined. There is no self-evident thing as a 'trait', a 'personality' a 'weak ego strength', 'self-awareness', 'emotional maturity', 'positive mental health', etc. These are words that are meant to help in dealing with certain problems, and can be only understood and measured if they are clearly defined, that is, the meaning of each of the concepts is what the measurement of that concept produces. This is an important factor to be taken into consideration, and any attempt to evaluate an intervention or assess the outcomes of a treatment will have to consider the definition of the aims and objectives.

As was stated earlier, the treatment will include a number of methods, so it will be important to organize them in a hierarchical order in terms of the learning process. Therefore, the necessary components must initially be established, and related to the chosen treatment.

The methods mainly in use in behaviour modification include certain aspects of social learning, such as modelling, as well as positive control and reinforcement of the changes in behaviour, aversive control (still in dispute), extinction, desensitisation, and so on. All these methods are complex and costly in terms of time and involvement, and it will require a professionally trained person to implement them.

There are, however, simpler methods which have been used by trained lay persons and which have shown a certain degree of success. They have been used in running anti-smoking clinics, weight reduction clinics, clinics for pregnant women and mothers with small babies, and others.

Training the trainers

People who run these clinics are usually partly trained lay persons with a medical, nursing, psychology or social work background. Their training courses last from a few days to several weeks or months. They may be for practitioners or trainers of practitioners. There are attempts to professionalise such activities, because at present there is very little control over the procedure or the outcomes. There are, however, a number of reputable educational institutions which have entered into this field of training and there is every possibility that the practitioners in the field of helping others will become professionally more accountable.

THE COMMUNITY APPROACH

Introduction

The concept of 'community' implies that there is a relatively large number of people living together and sharing certain values and interests, as well as interacting for a certain purpose or a shared goal. The concept of 'community' was originally used to denote rural settlements (villages) and now is used to denote a group of people sharing a location and common values and aims, such as an enterprise, school, city, and any other setting. The traditional 'community organization' approach has gradually evolved and the present form of this approach is very relevant to the new settings approach in health promotion and health education. It will be useful to explore certain aspects of the traditional community organization and community development approaches as compared to the new 'community participation' approach.

There is a difference between traditional community 'organization' and 'development' approaches as compared with the more recent community 'participation' or 'ecological' approach, as recommended by WHO. The traditional community development and community organization approaches have been concerned with a set of experts (agents of change) deciding what the community needs are (by observation, epidemiological studies or by mortality and morbidity statistics); this has then been followed by experts finding a 'key person' (or gate keeper) and selling the idea to him/her in the hope that he/she would be able to sell it to the community as a whole; once the community accepted the idea it was expected to provide support for the experts to carry out their intervention.

The ecological approach is based on community participation and includes the following steps:

- *needs definition* - which can be defined by scientific or epidemiological data, or based on the definition by the community members (felt needs);

- *enabling process* - which includes the selection of leaders, their training and support in achieving their goals; the leaders then carry out planning, definition of aims and objectives and they carry out the intervention as a long term process;

- *monitoring and evaluation* - which ensures the achievement of set goals, and through the feed-back mechanism, enables the correction of any negative side-effects.

In addition, working with communities involves adopting models which accord with current practices and values, following the diagnosis of community problems.

Health promotion and health education can use the community approach for two purposes: a community can be used for a health promotion and health education intervention or it can become a 'health promoting community' following the principles of 'health promoting settings', and integrating health promotion and health education into all the daily activities of such a community.

Community Participation

The 'community participation' method used by health promotion and health education has been developed and improved with the acceptance of the 'settings approach'. There are many similarities between the concept of a 'community' and a 'setting'. Applied in the field of health, the reinterpretation of the concept of community participation has moved away from the existing health education 'blame the victim' approach, and placed new demands on the methodology of health promotion and health education interventions.

The new approach is based on the interaction between external factors and community forces. It consists of two phases: the activities relating to external factors and those activities of the community, as shown in the following diagram.

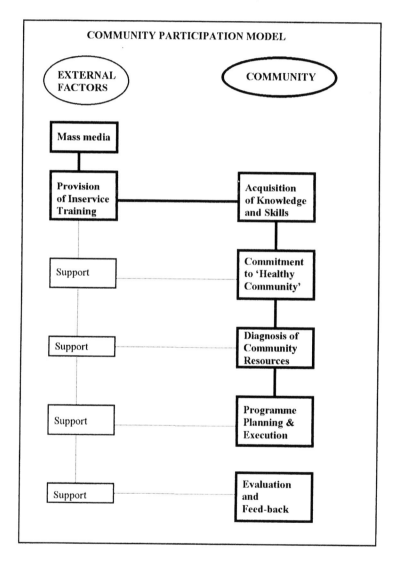

External Factors

1. On a local level an appropriate agency (health education, health promotion, health service, etc.) may develop a movement aimed at popularizing the concept of, for example, 'healthy' cities, enterprises, schools, hospitals or communities by using the media, and gaining support of important political representatives.

2. Once the idea becomes familiar and generally accepted, the appropriate agency creates and popularizes the fact that certain training facilities or workshops are available for those 'settings'leaders who are interested, where they can acquire competence in carrying out such programmes in their own settings (communities). The contents should be within the framework of health promotion, and include competence in dealing with different settings (community) problems of which health is only one aspect. The outcome should be that a number of leaders become involved in such learning ventures.

Settings (Community) Forces

1. The second phase is characterized by the shift of focus from the center into communities. On return from the learning venture, the local leader(s) or representatives, having acquired some competence, can discuss with other members the possibilities of taking on the commitment to nominate their community (or setting) as being 'healthy'.

2. Once general agreement has been reached and the commitment has been made, the preparations should be made for local leaders to take the first step in their own programmes.

3. The first step will be the assessment of community resources in terms of a multisectoral approach to the diagnosis of needs and planning, and the execution of solutions. The competence to carry out this kind of diagnosis should be a part of the training programme, and should allow for the necessary outside help and support.

4. The second step will be the development of an intervention programme including the role definition of the participants, distribution of resources, development of indicators for evaluation and a plan for action. There should be a set of short-term and long-term aims and objectives, which will form the basis for evaluation. In addition to acquired knowledge, outside help may be mobilised.

5. Evaluation should be a part of the intervention, with feed-back mechanisms allowing for the adjustments of the intervention. In addition to acquired knowledge, outside help may be mobilised.

This new interpretation of community participation in promoting members' own health is characterized by two types of activity which are clearly visible: that of the external factors, and that of the community. The roles of both are clearly defined and members of the community, within their own limits of available resources, do the actual work. Outside help is mainly concerned with raising the competence of community members to deal with their own problems.

It is much wider than the existing concepts of health education, and should be considered as a part of health promotion. This should be taken into account when planning workshops for community leaders, and be reflected in the contents provided.

Although the definition of health problems is still within a medical model, the general needs of the community are much wider, and competence includes the ways of dealing with all of these needs and not the health problems alone.

This approach does not usually have the same benefits as some externally organized interventions, and the question of motivation is often raised. Nevertheless, if the movement towards health improvement becomes a part of national policy and is widely publicised, then participating in it and rejoicing in its achievement may provide sufficient recognition and prestige for the leaders, as well as the community.

Introduction

Making use of mass media in health education was, in historical terms, one of the first methods used by formal health education. The early decades of this century saw not only the use of mass media, but also attempts to improve the effectiveness of this approach by means of research and evaluation (Leather et al., 1981; Ogilvy, 1983).

The Theoretical Framework

The theoretical basis for the mass media method includes a number of concepts and models, all of which have been used explicitly or implicitly by the health education agents. Some of these can be summarised as follows:

Models: KAP and Social Marketing

In the early years of this century, formal health education was concerned with health improvements among the underprivileged population groups, in developing countries, as well as developed countries. The initial fact-finding surveys showed that one of the most common characteristics shared by these groups was ignorance of health issues. Considering the size of the populations in question and the limited number of health education agents, an efficient as well as effective way of spreading knowledge appeared to be through mass media. Since this did not in fact produce the desired improvements in health, the approach was extended to include the development of positive attitudes, to accompany the newly gained knowledge.

After the Second World War, the researchers looking at health education practices developed the Knowledge-Attitude-Practice Model (KAP) as a framework for their research. The findings from studies of the application of this extended KAP model were not encouraging, and further developments followed. One of the side-effects of research into the KAP model, however, was improved insight into the use of mass media. This research is well documented, and includes comparative studies of lecture versus group discussions, the effectiveness of posters versus live lectures, and among others, prerequisites for efficient and effective exhibitions. With the further developments in health education, the KAP model fell into disrepute and was more or less abandoned. From time to time, someone came up with the idea of using the KAP model, to be immediately labelled as 'uninitiated' or even worse, 'ignorant' in terms of health education methodology.

Gradually new models were developed, stressing the advantages of individual and group approaches, with the consequence that the use of mass media fell into disrepute as an effective health education method. Everyone who was anyone in health education knew that knowledge did not mean action. This lasted for quite a while, until more recently, with the introduction of the Social Marketing Model, mass media came back into fashion.

The Social Marketing Model is in fact an approach based on the developments in marketing techniques, as a part of business studies. Originally relevant to commerce, by analogy it has been applied in health education under the assumption that health could also be treated as a marketable commodity.

Tones (1990) gives a very good description of this approach, and quotes Solomon on the ten key marketing concepts having relevance for health promotion through public health campaigns. These are:

- *'the marketing philosophy'*, which is based on the idea of 'exchange' and the prime role of satisfying consumer needs;

- *the four P's* (product, price, place, promotion), which are also known as the 'marketing mix'. This deals with the characteristics of the product; its price, which should be affordable, attractive and accessible; and places importance on advertising;

- the *'hierarchy of communication effects'*, which implies that one should take into account the fact that certain interventions can have short and long term effects, and that the indicators should be chosen to cover the whole range of the change process;

- the *'audience segregation'* principle, which is based on the assumption that targeted messages will be more effective than those aiming at the whole population, which is composed of different groups with different needs and characteristics;

- the *'understanding of the market'*, which is obviously a necessary precondition and implies that in addition to the consumer, other market forces may be present and affect the campaign;

- *'feed-back'*, which is a part of the evaluation process and should be used to adjust the programme during its development;

- *'interpersonal and mass communication interaction'*, which is concerned with the need to support mass media campaigns with personal educational programmes;

- *'commercial resources'* utilisation, which means that the field of health can benefit from the experiences of commercial expertise;

- *'competition'*, which is an important aspect of marketing, and has been increasingly important in the National Health Service.

- *'expectations'*, which must be defined if a campaign is to be evaluated, as is regularly done in commerce, where the accountability concerning expenditure and results has always had a high priority.

One of the most important aspects of the Social Marketing Model, which was obscured within the 'hierarchies, steps and rules' of the model, was the indirect reintroduction of mass media and advertising into health promotion and education.

It is now accepted, and to be expected, that money will be spent on advertising, as can be seen in the comprehensive advertising campaigns in the early days of AIDS. Not only is advertising a required part of health promotion, it is also permitted and expected that advertising agencies will be employed to promote both 'health' and the 'prevention' of certain risk factors, as if they were products.

Mass communication theories

Telling people what is best for them is not sufficient to reduce the prevalence of a health threat due to behaviour. The examination of various attempts to find an effective way of achieving this reduction supports this assumption. It has been shown, following Cohen (1964, 1972), that it is not theoretically correct to translate a population probability of a risk to its individual members. It has also been shown that, although individuals tend to do this all the time, the translation will depend on individual characteristics, value orientation, cultural and social background, etc. This indicates that it cannot be used as a practical tool for planning a health education approach aimed at individuals. It has been shown, furthermore, that individual perceptions of the probability of a health threat differ to such an extent, that no individual-based approach to a population could cover all the necessary variations. This has been supported by findings from mass health education campaigns, most of which have been effective only for a small proportion of a population. It should not be forgotten that nearly everybody in England knows about the risk smokers run from lung cancer and some other diseases, and yet only a small proportion of smokers (especially teenagers, and teenage girls) give it up in any one year. Even if smokers have attended some smoking clinics, where more intensive methods are being used, again only a small percentage continue to give it up for at least five years.

Studies in communication produced a new insight into the reasons why the transmission of information via mass media does not always work. The development of the 'two step' communication model explained the process of acquiring, internalising and acting upon information received by means of mass media. The model postulates that the crucial role in this process is played by 'gate keepers' or 'reference persons' or 'opinion leaders' in a certain field and in a certain community.

These mediators serve as sounding boards for new ideas, as models in adoption of innovations, and legitimisers of new social expectations. The outcome of this insight was that the mass media were considered as only one element in behavioural change, with the social support element playing a crucial role in activating the gained knowledge.

Implications for health promotion and education

This brings us back to the various ways in which health knowledge is transmitted and internalised. It would appear (Baric, 1976) that the most economical procedure for health education would be to influence routines and habits through the socialisation process, and at the same time to institutionalise at-risk statuses, together with the accompanying norms for each health threat. This is the way in which health education can operate successfully on a population level. Individuals who do not conform to social expectations (deviants) and other special cases can then be approached on an individual level by specially trained health educators and other professionals. In the case of new medical discoveries, it will also be more economical for health education to concentrate on the integration of this new knowledge into new norms, with sufficient power to act as a cue for individual action. In this way people could conform to well-defined social expectations related to health, instead of making haphazard individual choices which may produce unexpected and undesirable results.

As far as the mass media are concerned, it has been shown that they have a limited value in transmitting information on an individual level, as a means of producing an action or a change in behaviour. Their main advantage lies in the fact that they act on a 'mass' level and affect whole populations simultaneously. Thus, the mass media become vital in creating and affecting social norms, since this can only be achieved by transmitting information to whole populations at the same time.

The invention of printing, and the production of the first newspapers, started the mass communication revolution. The following technological developments such as radio, telegraph, telephone, photography, films, television, satellite communication, computer technology and multimedia, have brought about a radical change in the assessment of the impact of the mass media on human behaviour, their value system and their sharing of expectations. Its growth has resulted in a more personalised awareness of cultural differences, and produced a system of instant information, with the possibility of conceptualising earth as a planet with limited resources and humans as living in a 'global village'.

This new situation makes it difficult to apply relatively simplistic theories of mass communication (especially those developed in the field of health education) to a world in which, for example, hundred of millions of people could watch the horrors of a war in their sitting room every day, hear the noises and see the numbers of dead and wounded, not to mention witness the suffering of the civilian populations. Existing theories usually deal with one medium operating on a mass level (newspaper, television, etc.). The fact is that in the present situation we are part of a 'multi-media on a mass level' culture. The models and theories need to be much more complex to be able to account for the cultural differences within which multi-media mass communication operates.

Advertising

As we have already seen, advertising as a part of health promotion and education is aimed at selling the commodity called 'health'. Some people seem to confuse the concept of advertising with that of mass media communication and mass campaigns. One good way of learning about advertising is to study the activities of those who grew rich in the advertising industry, or who grew rich by using successful advertising to sell their products.

A famous advertising personality wrote a book on advertising, in which he gives simple and straightforward advice to people interested in the business of advertising. His main advice was to spend proportionally most of the time on research and learning about the product. If at the end of that period, certain aspects of the product are identified as favourable and able to be used to influence the public to buy it, one has the basis for a promising advertising approach (Ogilvy, 1983).

Good advertising need not be 'creative'; but merely interesting enough to sell the product. This interest aspect means that the successful advertisement uses the right 'appeal', which prompts consumers to buy a specific and not a generic product of the kind advertised. This implies that in advertising one is concerned with 'brand images', and 'brand loyalty' in the consumer. One should also bear in mind that any advertising that did not succeed in increasing the sales, might not be just 'unsuccessful', but could be actually harmful.

When everything that is to be known about the product has been learnt, the next step is to 'position' it, which means deciding which aspect of the product one will use in terms of 'what the product does and at whom is it aimed'. Positioning means choosing the right audience as the target for the advertisement and the right characteristics which will sell the product. It is clear that the images we have of many different products were created by the advertisers: the Volvo car as a 'winter' car, the VW Beetle as a reaction to vulgar big American petrol-guzzlers, the Marlboro as the macho cigarette. These are all examples of successful positioning of the product, and creating a niche for it in the market.

The next step is to decide on the 'brand' image. This is equivalent to the 'personality' of the product. It is a composition of its name, its packaging, its price, the style of its advertising and finally the nature of the product itself. There is an advantage in the continuation of the same image, although this is often impossible because of the change of the marketing director, the advertising agency or because the existing brand does not produce the expected results. There are situations in the market place which require a change in the brand image. For example in selling cars one can follow the change in brand image from a 'cheap' car to a 'cheap to run' car, to a 'reliable' car, to a 'green' car (using unleaded petrol with a catalytic converter). New scientific discoveries can also influence brand features, as in the case of sun lotions, from 'you will tan easily' to 'it protects you from skin cancer', combined with a whole supportive system of giving the protective value in numbers.

It is important to realise that a brand carries with it and sells an image. The image is created by advertising, but once it is created, it sells the product. One does not question the product, but the image that it represents. A very good example is the success of certain firms selling water. It seems impossible to make a fortune by bottling and selling ordinary drinking water. It was known that there was a lucrative market for 'mineral' water, which sold because of some 'health' property, but subsequently there was success in selling ordinary drinking water, such as the water from some undefined spring. It goes to show that one can sell anything with the right brand image. The macho image of Marlboro cigarettes has been stressed for 25 years, and only recently is being criticised as the result of increased public condemnation of the smoking habit.

The next step is to have 'a great idea', which will be proven great only if it sell the product. This is what the advertisers call the 'creative' part of the work, which differentiates between those who earn hundreds of thousands of pounds and those who loose their jobs after a few attempts. It is easy to recognise a good idea retrospectively, but very difficult to know in advance which idea is good. Long experience helps, although even the most successful advertisers remember those 'which got away'; and it does not help to rely solely on one's own feelings and instincts: the consumers may react quite differently to the same image.

The product should be made the 'hero' of the advertisement. There are no dull products, only dull writers. The problem with writers is that in addition to ideas they must have sufficient time to think out, test and produce an idea. This includes a considerable period of testing within the advertising agency, as well as within the organization that commissioned the advertisement. There is a tendency for writers to specialise in various professional activities, both in terms of background knowledge and of ideas.

There is some dispute about the possibility of evaluating an advertisement. There may be so many factors involved in selling a product that it is not possible to measure the contribution of the advertisement as such. Some cynics say that advertisers are only good at selling themselves and the idea of advertising to the customers, without any great impact on the selling of the product. People's awareness of the product and their opinions about the advertisements can be measured, and they can even be asked whether the advertisement influenced them in buying the product. People may say "yes", but in fact they themselves often do not exactly know why they bought something, and what part the advertisement played.

One of the questions that is often raised is associated with the selection of appeals to be used in selling a product. Great emphasis has been placed on the appeal of sex, and the role of fear. Whole books have been written on the advantages of certain appeals and preferential images such as children, young animals and nudes. Experience has shown that almost anything can be made acceptable if the purpose is acceptable, as was the case in the first use of condoms in advertisements about AIDS in the mass media.

Another means of learning about advertising is to see what the opposition does and, after a critical assessment, learn from their successes. Health education and promotion has been for some time in direct competition with tobacco manufacturers as far as advertising is concerned in their fight to abolish smoking. There have been numerous studies and publications based on the examination of cigarette advertisements; a number of laws and voluntary codes of practices have been adopted, and smoking is banned from an increasing number of places. To find out whether smoking is becoming less acceptable, it is necessary to look at the advertising agencies and their willingness to take on the tobacco industry as their clients. In general smoking is becoming less acceptable, but top advertisers proudly still display their successes in selling cigarettes, thanks to their advertisements. The reduction in smoking is in fact mainly a Western European and in part U.S. occurrence, while there is very little evidence of the reduction in smoking in Africa, Asia and Eastern Europe. Since most of tobacco industries are multinational, they can still spend millions on advertising and sponsoring world events, including until recently sport. There is, however, a growing tendency, especially among European countries, to ban tobacco advertising from sport.

It may seem inappropriate to speak in general terms about advertising in health promotion and education. Advertising is concerned with selling a product (cigarettes), and health promotion and health education are concerned with preventing people from buying and using it. This seems to be the main reason why it is difficult to translate experience from advertising and marketing to health promotion and health education. Another problem is that a topic may be subject to so many taboos that it is not possible to exploit all the experience learnt from other types of advertising, such as selling cosmetics. The latter is a very good example of selling images and illusions, supported by glamorous images and carefully phrased claims for the products. If one could use such tactics to sell condoms, maybe the use of condoms would increase, and thus contribute to the prevention of AIDS and unwanted pregnancies. In recent years, the AIDS campaigns have had a very high profile, and large amounts of money have been spent on advertising, but as was stated earlier, it is impossible to causally link any changes in behaviour, or in the prevalence of the infection, with the existing advertising campaigns, although it seems that AIDS is on the decrease. The same applies to unwanted pregnancies, which are on the increase among teenage girls. The question is whether the advertising has benefited more in promoting the institutions that spent the money on advertising, than in the prevention of disease, which should have been the main purpose.

Multi-media

The time in which we live may one day be labelled as the information society, since the advent of the microchip has revolutionised the way in which we communicate, interact, work and play. The first attempt at a mass application of the new technology in the field of education, started with such activities as television programmes as a part of the Open University 'education for the masses' approach, followed by the distribution of computers in classrooms, and the spread of 'computer literacy' among the new generations of children in this country.

Health education, and later health promotion, followed this information and communication technology revolution and tried to keep abreast of the new developments. It started in the early days with the 'Radio Doctor' programmes, as a special feature aimed at informing people about new medical developments, and became a true 'multisectoral activity', with widespread use of health as news items, scientific topics, political issues, contents of soap operas, advertising appeals, etc.

The combination of interactive audio and visual communication with broad based networks, as well as television and video recorders has resulted in the development of a potentially effective learning method in the form of 'multimedia technology', which is a combination of technologies which allows the mixture of computer-generated text, graphics and animations, live and still video images and sound. As a new technology, it provided new and cheaper tools for video production, video-graphics, music, animation, advertising and business presentations. The I nternet is a source of huge amounts of data. Development in this field is rapid, with multimedia, interactive video, simulation and virtual reality increasingly used for training purposes, from teaching workers technical skills, to training managers how to manage multi-national corporations. There are now programmes for training professionals such as doctors in various skills related to medical diagnosis and interventions as well as surgical skills.

Although health education and promotion have not as yet been able to make full use of the newest information technology on a large scale, the learning videos have been highly successful in enabling people to become familiar with various health topics, such as first aid, looking after a new baby, reducing weight, exercising, relaxing, etc.

The whole concept of 'mass media' has changed from media which transmit messages on a mass scale, to media which are being used by masses of people on an individual basis in their homes, or as part of individual learning programmes in schools (every student with his/her own computer).

The multi-media revolution has led to the growth of new professions or experts for different media, and to new and different uses of the same media. There are increasing numbers of specialist firms that deal with the preparation and production of the new media, or programmes for the new applications of the more conventional media. An important development is the growth of 'in-house' experts, as in the case of desk-top publishing, which is a part of many health promotion and health education units.

Another important aspect of the availability of the new technology is the software that is being developed in the fields of data collection (databases), analysis (spreadsheets) and communication (word processing) for existing personal computers. Various data-base programs facilitate the storage of whole libraries of information with easy and immediate access; there are statistical packages, which enable in-house analysis of survey data from quite large samples; other management programs allow for the analysis of future trends and can accommodate simulation models, together with graphical animation programs; other developments enable networking and direct links with other computers and access to their data as in the case of access to different libraries in the world. The access to Internet has extended the available information even more although it is still in its infancy as far as health promotion and health education are concerned. All this technology could represent a qualitative jump in the performance of health education and promotion units once its potential is fully exploited. It is becoming increasingly obvious that the life-style of people is changing, as a result of the developments in information technology. People learn, think, make decisions, and are entertained differently as the result of this technological revolution. Health promotion and education must take these developments into account if it does not want to lose touch with the current transformation.

165

Among the population in general there is a growing concern about and interest in health issues. In the early days of health education, people depended for expert information on the activities of health education specialists who were paid to transmit information about diseases and their prevention. With the growth of information technology, direct on-line access to information has become widespread. The business of providing health information has exploded, with endless books and videotapes on staying healthy, beautiful, young, slim and attractive, as well as Internet sites dealing with the latest developments in medical knowledge.

The differentiation between health education and health promotion and the emphasis on the settings approach have resulted in the inclusion of a range of people and professions into these activities. This has raised the question of the protection of consumers. It is increasingly important to keep abreast of these developments and to learn from the accumulated experience.

Currently, the issue of **accountability** is at the forefront of these developments, both because of the variety of people and professions practising HP/HE and because of increasing sophistication in the expectations of the consumers.

In this paper I wish to address this issue by tracing briefly the history of the way people have dealt with accountability in the past and looking towards future trends:

The historical developments

The main characteristic of the early period was *'hoping for the best'*, where the activity of preventing disease and improving health was based on the transmission of information (the cognitive model) and the responsibility lay with consumers to make the best use of the information received. Improvements largely lay in the sophistication of methods of transmitting information and dealing with the barriers that reduced effectiveness.

The call for accountability arose largely from the demands of fund givers who wanted to know how the money had been spent. This resulted in the development of **evaluation methods** concerned with monitoring the activities in terms of the effort rather than effectiveness of the transmission process. Such evaluation went through a process of clarification and increased scientific rigour through differentiating its various aspects (process vs. outcome; effectiveness, efficiency, and effort; and so on) and through making explicit the necessary parameters (aims, objectives, methods, indicators, and criteria). The main overall characteristic of evaluation was that it was **carried out after the completion of the intervention,** and that it ideally measured the achievement of the stated aims of an intervention.

The shift of emphasis to people with problems who live, work and play in various settings (the organizational model) has resulted in recognising the need for the accountability of people, within settings, who are engaged in HP/HE activities. There have been attempts to introduce external evaluation of HP/HE activities into various settings (schools, hospitals, enterprises, and so on), that have either met with resistance or outright rejection by the people working in these settings.

A more recent development has been to utilise the existing monitoring mechanisms in such settings, such as the **quality management systems**, and to add health indicators to the existing specifications of each setting. This has required the understanding of quality management, the design of health specifications and the ways of measuring the outcomes. The most important aspect of this approach has been that it took place **during the process of intervention** and allowed for corrections and adjustments, thus ensuring a positive outcome.

The new approach

The ever-greater demand for accountability has further extended the scope of evaluation from the justification of expenditure of resources to include cost-benefit analysis and the protection of the human rights of the consumers. A new conceptual framework is here presented, which includes all the various methods of measurement relevant to HP/HE activities and interventions set out in a sequential order:

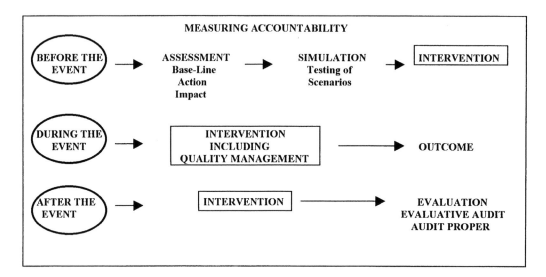

Before the event: During the planning stages it is necessary to introduce the process of assessment, which includes the following aspects:

> *Base-line assessment* - which establishes the characteristics of the environment and the actors involved in the planned activity;

> *Action assessment* – which considers the various methods available for the planned activity;

Impact assessment – which translates the planned activities within a defined environment into scenarios, and by using simulation methods, establishes the optimal scenario for the planned activity.

During the event: The intervention process is embedded in *quality management*, which assures that the quality of each step in the process meets pre-defined specifications, and thus reduces the risk of any negative outcomes.

After the event: The achievements of the intervention can be measured in various ways:

Evaluation –this measures the achievement of the pre-defined aims of an intervention through attention to defined objectives (methods), indicators and criteria;

Evaluative audit –this takes place when the intervention has been carried out without clearly defined aims, objectives, indicators and criteria, but an outcome can be measured against expectations, which can be defined by stakeholders, consumers or can be a part of general norms;

Audit proper – this can be carried out by external authorised agents, where the process and the outcome are measured against already established external norms (legal, financial, professional, and so on).

The methods of measuring what is planned, of choosing the best fit through simulation methods, measuring the process and finally the outcome, should set new standards for the practice of HP/HE and answer the demands for the accountability of the various formally recognised agents active in this field. The activities of the many informal agents, however, can only be audited and the results used as a basis for possible litigation depending on the potential harm caused to the consumers.

In brief, it can be said that people who are paid to carry out certain activity (directly or indirectly) should be held accountable for the process and the outcome of what they are doing to the consumers. Introducing explicit and scientifically defensible methods of monitoring and measurement is the only way to ensure this.

The differentiation between health promotion and health education has resulted in the need for different methods and indicators to ensure the accountability of planned policies and actions.

Health promotion is concerned with environmental factors (including physical and social environment) and deals with social structures, mechanisms and processes aimed at improving the health of a population. It will, therefore, require indicators that are appropriate for monitoring and recording events on a societal level. Health education is concerned with individual and small group factors (including the fact that people take on the responsibility for their own health) and deals with individual and group characteristics, competence and equity in the participatory processes of health improvement. The indicators will include the measurement and monitoring of group dynamics and the assessment of individual competence.

At present, health promotion activities depend on the political and professional definitions of problems and the solutions in the form of policy and strategy interventions. For example, on the international level, the WHO Ottawa Charter is a policy document, which has had very far-reaching implications for the practice of health promotion and health education in the world. On a national level, the UK Government produced a policy and strategy document *The New NHS* and a discussion document *Our Healthier Nation*. In both cases, the implications for the delivery of health care and the health of the population on international and national levels have been considerable. Systematic and scientific assessment, including base line, action and impact assessment for WHO documents is desirable, and in fact *Our Healthier Nation* does include a section on 'Health Impact Assessment'.

The main advantage of an assessment before an intervention takes place is that, by using systems or simulation methods, it is possible to develop a number of possible scenarios, select the optimal one according to the needs of the consumers and the resources of the intervention agents, and then translate it into an intervention.

It is possible to differentiate between three kinds of assessment. One is the assessment of certain institutions and organization and examines them as a part of a wider social system looking at their structural and functional characteristics in relationship to planned activities and possible changes ('base line assessment'). The second is the assessment of the interventions in terms of their chosen approach within a recognised theoretical framework and based on a 'differential diagnosis' of the needs ('action assessment'). The third is the assessment of the consequences of the actions, which include different policies and interventions ('Impact Assessment').

171

BASE LINE ASSESSMENT

To find out about a HP/HE intervention within a setting it is necessary to understand the environment in which the setting is located. At the same time, the setting as such needs to be defined as the environment in which people live, work and play and in which HP/HE activities are taking place. Since the concept of a setting is very general and can cover everything from a city or a multinational enterprise to a single-handed general practice or a family, it will be necessary to establish the base line characteristics of the setting derived from the environment in which it is located. These environmental characteristics relevant to HP/HE activities can be listed as follows:

Environmental Aspects	Service factors	Population aspects	HP/HE
Location Size Housing Commerce Transport Communication Employment, Etc.	Political Religious Social Legal Educational Health, Etc.	Density Race Religion Age Sex Family Income Education Health, Etc.	Health related behavior Health directed behavior Health interventions

These aspects and factors will provide the data, which will need to be translated into information about the characteristics of a setting relevant for a HP/HE intervention. It is easy to understand the large scale cultural differences between schools located in different regions and countries, and the mentioned aspects and factors should provide the kind of data necessary to establish the contribution of these aspects and factors to the assessment process relevant for HP/HE purposes.

Collection of information

The collection of data needs to be defined in terms of aims and objectives, such as:

Environmental factors

AIM 1: to establish the main physical characteristics of the setting in question; to achieve this aim the inquiry will have the following objectives:

Objective 1.1: to collect information about the location of the setting;

> *Indicator 1.1.1:* urban or rural location of the main office;
> *Indicator 1.1.2:* urban or rural location of branch offices, factories, workshops, warehouses, surgeries, classrooms, departments, etc.;
> *Indicator 1.1.3:* physical, social, cultural characteristics of the location;

Objective 1.2: to collect information about the size and the structure of the setting;

> *Indicator 1.2.1:* size in terms of number of subsidiaries, employees, consumers, etc.;
> *Indicator 1.2.2:* organizational and power structure of the setting;

Objective 1.3: to collect information about the type of the setting:

> *Indicator 1.3.1:* part of the production, distribution or service industry;
> *Indicator 1.3.2:* past history and prosperity, stability of employment;

Objective 1.4: to collect information about accessibility of the setting and communications:

> *Indicator 1.4.1:* access by employees;
> *Indicator 1.4.2:* access by customers, patients, pupils, etc.
> *Indicator 1.4.3:* communication technology (telephone, fax, email, web pages, etc.)

Service factors

AIM 2: to establish the main factors related to the activities of the setting with respect to the employees, consumers and the people in the community; to achieve this aim the inquiry will have the following objectives:

Objective 2.1: to find out about the top management of the setting concerning their agenda;

> *Indicator 2.1.1:* policy statements of the top management concerning their agenda;
> *Indicator 2.1.2:* relevance of the agenda to the health of the members of the setting;
> *Indicator 2.1.3:* special programmes concerning HP/HE;

Objective 2.2: to find out about the satisfaction of the employees or members of the setting;

> *Indicator 2.2.1:* the level of satisfaction concerning their work;
> *Indicator 2.2.2:* the level of satisfaction concerning their accommodation;
> *Indicator 2.2.3:* the level of satisfaction concerning their job security;

Objective 2.3: to find out about the satisfaction of consumers;

> *Indicator 2.3.1:* the level of satisfaction with the products;
> *Indicator 2.3.2:* the level of satisfaction with services;
> *Indicator 2.3.3:* the level of satisfaction with general treatment;

Objective 2.4: to find out the position of the setting within wider community;

> *Indicator 2.4.1:* the level of contribution of the setting to the community;
> *Indicator 2.4.2:* the strength of links with the community (alliances);
> *Indicator 2.4.3:* the effects of the setting on the environment;

Population aspects

AIM 3: to establish the various population characteristics of the management, employees, consumers and the wider community, which could be relevant for the success of HP/HE activities within a setting; to achieve this aim the inquiry will have the following objectives:

Objective 3.1: to look at population aspects within the mentioned groups concerning the density, religion, race, sex, age;

> *Indicator 3.1.1:* the size and distribution of the population;
> *Indicator 3.1.2:* predominant religion and religious relationships;
> *Indicator 3.1.3:* question of discrimination due to race , sex, age;

Objective 3.2: to look at the occupation, income and education within the mentioned population groups;

> *Indicator 3.2.1:* employment and social class distribution;
> *Indicator 3.2.2:* economic status within the population groups;
> *Indicator 3.2.3:* literacy and educational level within the population groups;

Objective 3.3: to look at the family composition and stages of development within the mentioned population groups;

> *Indicator 3.3.1:* predominant pattern of family composition and stage of development;
> *Indicator 3.3.2:* the number, age and position of children within the setting;
> *Indicator 3.3.3:* level of care for children, handicapped and elderly available;

Objective 3.4: to look at the levels of health and health care with respect to the mentioned population groups;

> *Indicator 3.4.1:* morbidity and mortality rates;
> *Indicator 3.4.2:* access to health care within the setting and within the community;
> *Indicator 3.4.3:* specific risk factors associated with the location, occupation, transport and personal behaviour of each of the mentioned population groups;

Health promotion and health education

AIM 4: to establish the existing and planned health promotion and health education activities within the setting; to achieve this aim the inquiry will have the following objectives:

Objective 4.1: to look at HP/HE activities relevant to the health related behaviour within the setting;

> *Indicator 4.1.1:* any existing projects or actions within the setting;
> *Indicator 4.1.2:* any existing projects or actions within the community;

Objective 4.2: to look at HP/HE activities relevant to health directed behaviour;

> *Indicator 4.2.1:* any activities associated with specific health problems;
> *Indicator 4.2.2:* any activities related to creating a health promoting setting;

Objective 4.3: to look at existing HP/HE interventions;

> *Indicator 4.3.1:* interventions within the setting;
> *Indicator 4.3.2:* interventions as part of the health promoting setting.

Interpretation of data

The collected data will need to be translated into information, which will enable the planning and execution of HP/HE interventions within a setting.

AIM 1 should provide information about the specific conditions, which need to be taken into consideration in the planning process. The type of location will decide what resources are available, what problems have to be solved and what advantages or disadvantages different types of interventions will have to solve.

AIM 2 should provide information about the characteristics of the setting, which will decide what possibilities and requirements the setting provides, what are the commitments of the management, and the needs of the personnel. All this should be translated into the possible contributions of the setting to the community in which the setting is located.

AIM 3 should provide information about the community from which the personnel is recruited and what problems need to be tackled by HP/HE.

AIM 4 should provide information about the possibilities that the existing HP/HE systems provides for tackling the problems within the setting as well as the problems within the community, affected by the setting.

All this information should be translated into HP/HE actions, which can then take the form of specific interventions.

ACTION ASSESSMENT

Answers to the following questions are involved in the assessment of any action relevant to health promotion and health education:

- What is being done?
- Why it is being done in this particular way?

The intervention

The description of an intervention ('what is being done') will include the different aspects of both a health promotion and a health education intervention. The methods used in health promotion will include the influence on the environment (both physical and social), and those used in health education will be directed toward individuals (including competence, coping and their adjustment to the environment).

The choice of methods will be based on 'differential diagnosis' as the justification for the selected methods of approach. This differential diagnosis will be carried out referring to the environmental as well as personal factors of the target population or targeted individuals. It will take into consideration all the available health promotion and health education methods and select those most appropriate (or most promising) for achievement of the health gain of the consumers (populations, communities, families, and individuals).

Differential diagnosis for health promotion and health education purposes is based on the experiences gained in medical differential diagnosis. It includes the consideration of a number of possible factors associated with a health threat or a health threatening behaviour, which are gradually reduced by elimination of the irrelevant ones or those that cannot be influenced by health promotion and health education interventions, to a limited number of those which can be influenced and subsequently integrated into the aims of the intervention.

The theoretical base

A highly qualified and experienced professional in health promotion and health education will be able to carry out a differential diagnosis of a problem situation and chose appropriate methods of intervention. Such a professional will chose the appropriate method(s) based on the theoretical knowledge gained during the educational process in achieving the recognised status of an expert. This theoretical knowledge should answer the question "why is something done?" in addition to the question "how is something done?"

Many theories relevant to health promotion activities, including sociological, management and social psychological theories. Other theories are relevant to health educational interventions, including those which focus on personality, decision-making, behaviour modification, learning, marketing, advertising, application of new technologies, etc.

IMPACT ASSESSMENT

Impact assessment is a part of a wider movement concerned with predicting possible outcomes in a number of areas such as Environmental Impact Assessment, Technology Assessment, Economic Impact Assessment, etc. One area is that of Social Impact Assessment (SIA), which is the closest to the needs of health promotion and health education assessment. It should be noted that so far there has been no attempt to develop a specific HP/HE Impact Assessment and SIA is being used as an example of what the development of an impact assessment method should include. SIA is a well-established method (Becker, 1997, Burdge, 1994(a), 1994(b), Burdge & Robertson, 1994, Canter, 1996, Coile, 1986, Finsterbusch & Wolf, 1981, Taylor, Bryan, & Goodrich, 1990, Twomey & Tomkins, 1993) which is designed to explore and predict the possible impact of various policies and actions.

The SIA operates on three levels: the *micro-level* (analysing impacts on behaviour of large numbers of individuals, as in demographic impact assessment), the *meso-level* (analysing impacts on the behaviour of collective authors, such as organizations and social movements) and the *macro-level* (analysing impacts on societal macro-systems, such as national and international political and legal systems). The steps in carrying out a SIA (Becker, 1997, p.87) include:

Step 1.0 Scenario design

      1.1 Choice of the type of scenarios to be designed
      1.2 Design of models
      1.3 Design of scenarios
      1.4 Design of critical incidents
      1.5 Iteration and reporting

Step 2.0 Design of strategies

      2.1 Evaluation of current strategies
      2.2 Design of an integrated set of strategies
      2.3 Iteration and reporting

Step 3.0 Assessment of impacts

      3.1 Scenario-to-strategy simulation
      3.2 Additional simulations
      3.3 Iteration and reporting

Step 4.0 Ranking of strategies

      4.1 Choice of type of ranking
      4.2 Ranking process
      4.3 Iteration and reporting

Step 5.0 Migration of negative impacts

    5.1 Redesigning of strategies and reassessment of impacts
    5.2 Revision of ranking strategies
    5.3 Iteration and reporting

Step 6.0 Reporting

    6.1 Decision about the types of reporting
    6.2 Executive summary
    6.3 Full report
    6.4 Background papers
    6.5 Press release
    6.6 Workshops

Step 7.0 Simulation of implementation

Step 8.0 Auditing and ex-post evaluation

    8.1 Auditing
    8.2 Ex-post evaluation

This brief description of SIA is aimed at informing decision-makers about available methods of benefit in the planning of policy and strategy of HP/HE. It should also enable the decision-makers and intervention agents to use the simulation approach to 'test' their policies and strategies in advance by simulating the system and gaining insight into potential outcomes without the need to find out about the impact after the event.

Health promotion and health education in settings operate within an organizational framework and need to take into account the methods and mechanisms for the assessment of the processes and outcomes already existing in a setting. An increasing number of formal settings carry out assessments through their quality management systems (QMS).

There are three ways that the principles of quality management can be used as a method of assessing HP/HE activities within settings:

- Utilization of an existing quality management system in a setting by adding health issues into the existing specifications;

- Introduction of QMS into a HP/HE institution followed by an application for certification from a recognized certifying body (such as ISO or BS or any other) and thus ensuring the quality of their activities in this field;

- Development of a specific QMS for HP/HE with appropriate standards and specifications and creating a new international certifying body for quality assessment of HP/HE in a Health Promoting Setting.

There is a growing demand for quality management in health promoting settings, which is the result of the increased demand for accountability of the providers of services. The possibility of harming the consumer (i.e. the patient) is widely recognized and often ends in litigation, with the patients suing the health service. In such cases, a detailed documentation of the procedures that have been implemented could serve as a protection for the health care staff. For this reason, as well as others, an increasing number of health care settings are introducing quality management systems. It is possible to envisage that all health care settings will in the future have such a system of monitoring the processes and outcomes of their activities.

Existing Quality Assessment

The emphasis now placed on settings has resulted in the introduction of an organizational model and extended the possibilities of assessment of HP/HE activities, through considering the reinforcement of evaluation by the existing quality management system of a setting. The idea of introducing HP/HE specifications into the existing quality assessment mechanisms represents an innovation that has not so far been empirically tested and justified. The description of the practical steps in introducing HP/HE into a quality management system of a health promoting setting represents an experiment, intended to explore this method of monitoring and assessing the activities of a setting.

To be able to use such an approach requires a full understanding of the existing quality management system. It requires a modification of the existing standards and specifications, in order to apply the principles of quality management to the assessment of HP/HE programme, without necessarily applying for a new certification of a quality management system by an external body. In general, it can be concluded that the introduction of HP/HE into the standards and specifications of an existing quality management system could represent a considerable improvement in the understanding of both processes and outcomes. This also applies to a specific type of quality assessment known as Total Quality Management (TQM), which uses a systems approach.

One of the first attempts to use TQM for the assessment of health promotion activities was carried out within the framework of 'Health Promoting Hospitals' in Vienna, Austria (Ernst & Stroheim, 1997). The Viennese Hospital Association developed TQM in four hospitals and two nursing homes, and the process is still being tested. The 'Health Promoting Hospital' movement is considering using this development as a part of their modified assessment procedure concerning the HP/HE activities within hospitals.

Seeking certification

Another way of using the principles of quality management in HP/HE is to introduce the QMS into the existing health promoting institutions. It should, however, be recognized that the introduction of QMS into an institution is a highly formalized procedure governed by strict rules and will require recognition in the form of certification from a recognized certifying body. It should also be recognized that there is a difference in the terminology used by existing evaluation procedures and QMSs. There have already been instances where the concept of quality management has been seen as contributing to the improvement of the delivery of HP/HE services and some HP/HE Units have considered introducing it into their work. One such instance of achieving certification is the 'ISO 9000' Health Mark Award for provision of training and library services for the Health Promotion Department, Westcare Business Services, Londonderry, N.Ireland (O'Doherty, 1997). Other attempts have been made to introduce quality management into HP/HE based on the Health Education Authority's publication *Assuring Quality in Health Promotion* (Evans, Head & Speller, 1994). The approach recommended is a mixture of evaluation and QMS, with interchangeable terminology, but without provision for seeking a formal certification.

A successful introduction of quality management into HP/HE institutions will require an understanding of the conditions and procedures involved in carrying out QMS and acquiring certification from a recognized authority.

Standards

The assessment of the quality of a product or service will only be possible if the expected and acceptable quality of the services provided can be defined. These expectations can be expressed in a set of standards and specifications.

The concept of 'standards' has a specific meaning when related to the idea of measuring performance in terms of quality. In this context *standards apply to the requirements for the introduction and management of the quality assessment system in a setting*. It is not directly related to the quality of the product. These requirements are in general defined by a number of national or international bodies that are recognized as having the authority to certify such a quality assessment system in a setting. The standards are, therefore, only indirectly related to the quality of the product, but are directly related to the administrative system required for the monitoring and assessment of quality in a setting.

There are various ways the quality of a product or a service can be assessed. The method will depend on the conceptual framework used in defining the meaning of quality.

Quality has been considered as an expression of excellence and meeting some high specifications; it has been used to characterize consistency, fitness for purpose, value for money, meeting the expectations of the fund-giving bodies or as a means of transformation. In more general terms, quality is *'meeting the requirements of the customer'*. In educational terms it needs to be recognized that in any process there will be a whole set of 'qualities' which will have to be met in order to satisfy the needs of the consumer. This multiplicity of qualities will be of special importance in the case of a setting approach to health promotion and health education, with each setting having different specifications and consequently different qualities to be measured.

The role of external consultants

The introduction of a Quality Management System (QMS) into a setting is a complex procedure and has been the area of expertise of accredited management specialists, who act as external consultants to a setting. Their role is even more important if a setting aims at obtaining certification.

Within the general framework of the role of consultants (Hope, 1992) the specific role of a consultant as an enabler for a setting to introduce a QMS will consist of the following support:

- explanation of the requirements and advantages of a QMS for that setting;
- training of different levels of management in carrying out the necessary activities (preparing a policy statement, developing a QMS structure, meeting the required standards, specifications and procedures);
- establishment of documentation systems for quality assessment;
- role definition of various actors.

The consultants will act as a bridge between the setting and the certifying body and aim to ensure the success of the application for certification when all the standards are fulfilled. The consultant in some cases may be also an accredited assessor for the certifying body and be responsible for yearly monitoring of the activities in the light of the requirements of a QMS.

Certification

The introduction of a QMS into a service provider organization should produce a competitive edge in a market economy. This can only be achieved if such a quality driven service is visible and formally recognized or *certified*. This can be achieved by registration with respect to a specific Quality System Standard such as for example the early BS 5750. The accredited assessment body should be consulted in choosing the appropriate Standard. There are a number of accredited bodies, some of which are specialized (for example UK Certification Authority for Reinforcing Steels - CARES) where others are of a more general character (for example British Standard Institute Quality Assurance - BSI, or Lloyds Register Quality Assurance Ltd - LRQA).

The concept of certification has been increasingly gaining in importance. This is especially the case in industry, where the idea has become so widespread that it may soon be only possible to compete as a supplier if an organization is certified for quality. In the service industry this is also becoming increasingly important, where the purchasers of services may favor providers of services certified for quality.

This will not necessarily be the case, however, since management movements come and go, and there is no doubt that the quality movement has been somewhat of a crusade in management. Nevertheless, the concepts and procedures underlying quality management are so important that the shifts of fashion should leave its common sense core untouched. For health promotion and health education, its importance lies in encouraging the introduction of QMS into health planning, delivery of health services and health promotion and health education interventions while making sure that quality management systems should, wherever possible, incorporate health promotion and health education aspects.

The introduction to ISO 9004 establishes the involvement of the members of the organization to ensure the necessary quality of the services provided:

- managing the social processes involved in the service;
- regarding human interactions as a crucial part of the service quality;
- recognizing the importance of a customer's perception of the organization's image, culture and performance;
- developing the skills and capability of the personnel;
- motivating personnel to improve quality and to meet customer expectations.

The requirements for certification are set out in each Standard and can be summarized as follows:

- quality must be management led: it has to include the understanding and meeting of customer needs; the understanding of the business processes; and investing time and effort to prevent errors;

- only senior managers can change the philosophy and the culture of the organization; they must ensure that the aims are understood by everyone; they must demonstrate their commitment in actions and words; they must encourage the full participation of all the employees in the efforts of achieving quality of services;

- the management has five key roles: (i) determine the aims of the business, its philosophy and policy for quality; (ii) develop the QMS to ensure this policy is understood and implemented at all levels; (iii) encourage every employee to become involved in implementing the QMS; (iv) invest in the necessary skills and resources to ensure the QMS is effective; and (v) take an active role in implementing and developing QMS.

BS 5750

The main principle of BS 5750 which was the first widely used standard, is that the set of standards should meet the needs and the interests of the organization, as well as meeting the needs and expectations of customers.

The management should be responsible for introducing this system by setting out its policy, based on consultations with members of staff and taking into account the interests of the clients.

The implementation of the quality management system should ensure that the objectives related to quality are satisfied. The emphasis should be on problem prevention rather than problem detection after occurrence.

The management should plan and measure the quality related costs concerning the introduction and management of the quality system, as well as possible changes and improvements in the production process.

The management should introduce quality aspects into marketing, specifications and design, procurement, production and control of production, product verification. It should also be concerned with the measurement control, nonconformity and coercive action. Management should plan and control handling and post-production functions, quality documentation and control, personnel training, product safety and liability, and should be able to use statistical methods for the implementation of quality control systems.

Performance indicators need to be related to the objectives of the organization under consideration. They can be broken down into input, process and output indicators and may also be categorized in terms of efficiency, effectiveness and economy. All performance indicators need to be related to the different types of interests of the stakeholders. In educational institutions, performance indicators for teaching and learning may include graduate destinations, degree classifications, value added, wastage and completion rates and student evaluations.

An important factor in the assessment of an educational institution is peer review, which can take three main forms: reputational studies, external examining and peer review based on a visit by a team.

Another way of assessing the performance of an educational institution is by inspection, which can include inspection surveys as well as informal inspections.

The certification of a quality management system in a setting, such as for example, an educational setting when applying the BS 5750 standards, will require that the setting meets the following preconditions:

- production of a quality policy document signed by the top management of the setting;
- definition of the role of the personnel related to quality management including their responsibilities and their authority;
- verification of the resources and personnel, which includes monitoring the services and defining the resources for the implementation of quality assessment;
- selecting a management representative and his deputy with the responsibility for managing the quality assessment system;
- carrying out a management review with special reference to the quality system introduced; the required documentation; concern about purchaser satisfaction; publishing of the examination results; and the design of programmes related to the production process;
- control of the quality system with special reference to its functions; relevant factors; relevant activities; other factors affecting quality;
- review of the contracts, which should include the factors related to the purchaser-provider interface, enrolment of staff, introduction of processes assuring quality and the methods of assessment of the outcomes;
- design control which should be reflected in the planning and the development of programmes; definition of methods; selection of contents and building in of mechanisms necessary for peer or government reviews;
- document control which is related to the relevant quality issues; which should be approved by the certifying body; and which should include possibilities for modifications or changes;
- purchasing, which should be related to the defined specifications; it should be carried out from assessed sources; it should define contractors and sub-contractors; and it should include the verification of products;
- product identification and traceability which should be reflected in the documentation concerning quality management;
- general and special process control which should include course planning, development, evaluation and review; timetabling; attendance; delivery; AV aids; accommodation; facilities; library;
- inspection, which should be concerned with incoming consumers; in-process inspection; final inspection and testing, as well as inspection of test records;
- equipment, which will include the inspection, measurement and testing of the equipment used; its condition and the appropriate inspections and tests;
- control of the product; with special reference to non-conforming products, services and the character of this non-conformity;
- corrective action which includes the mechanisms for complaints and comments, results of audit, as well as retention and success rates based on the analysis of the process;
- handling, storage, packaging and delivery of products which in an educational institution refers to student/trainee care, available instructions and health care, counselling, personal safety, accommodation and lodgings, etc.;
- quality records, which should include student and staff records;
- audit, which should be carried out internally and by external auditors; and which should be concerned with the training processes;

- training of staff, which includes the induction process, staff development and extensions, possibilities for retraining; mechanisms for staff relationship with the management through the process of communication;
- servicing of the institution which will include contract agreements, as well as support by students after completing their training;
- statistical techniques, which will be required for the analysis of performance indicators; drop-out rates; achievement records; purchaser satisfaction; as well as identifying the future trends in the institutional development.

Implementation of QMS - The management responsibilities

The decision within a setting to integrate health promotion and health education into daily activities will imply the introduction of a quality management system (QMS) into the monitoring and evaluation of the setting's activities. The main characteristic of a QMS in a service industry is that the focal point in the system is the customer. It also includes the management responsibilities and the personnel and material resources as well as the quality management structure.

The quality policy

The management is responsible for the provision of services to the customers. For this purpose it has to design a policy for satisfying the customers' needs and expectations. If the provision of services is based on the concept of quality, then the management has to undertake a commitment to quality management and introduce a *quality management system (QMS)*.

This commitment will be expressed in the *quality policy*, which has to be produced by the top management. The quality policy will include:

- the service organisation's image and reputation for quality;
- the type of service to be provided (specifications);
- the objectives for the achievement of service quality (procedures);
- the approaches or methods used for the achievement of quality objectives; and
- the role of personnel responsible for implementing the quality policy.

Quality aims and objectives

The achievement of quality policy will require a clear statement of the *aims* or goals of the service organization, such as:

- effectiveness leading to customer satisfaction and consistent with professional standards and ethics;
- continuous monitoring and improvement of services;
- adjusting services to the needs of the society and the environment;
- efficiency in providing the services.

The achievement of these quality aims will depend on the selection of *objectives or specifications* including the following activities:

- clear definition of the customer's needs which should include appropriate indicators and criteria related to quality assessment;
- application of appropriate procedures related to aims;
- preventive actions to avoid customer dissatisfaction;
- optimising quality-related cost for the required performance and type of service;
- continuous review of service requirements and achievements to identify opportunities for service quality improvement;
- preventing adverse effects of the service activities on the society and the environment.

Quality responsibility and authority

The achievement of the stated aims through the selected objectives requires the establishment of a *quality system structure* to carry out effective evaluation and control of service quality intended to result in possible improvements.

The purpose of such a quality system structure is to provide a picture of the distribution of authority and role definition (job description) of the personnel in accordance with the requirements of the provision of services. The system should pay special attention to the qualitative and quantitative aspects of the personnel-supplier relationship at all interfaces within and external to the organization.

Top management needs to ensure the development and smooth operation of the requirements for a quality system. The responsibility should be allocated to a *special person* or form a part of the overall role of a person. It is important, however, to understand the holistic character of the quality management approach. Quality depends not only on a designated person or on the performance of a part of the role of a person. It is the outcome of a *total commitment and aggregated performance* of all personnel, expressed in their commitment, motivation, involvement and networking. The main theme, however, is continuous improvement of services.

Management review

Management should make provision for *formal, periodic and independent review* of the quality system and their own responsibilities for its implementation, with a view to possible improvement. It should include a well structured and comprehensive *evaluation* based on the following information:

- findings of a service performance analysis: i.e. information on the overall effectiveness and efficiency of the service delivery process in achieving service requirements and customer satisfaction;
- findings of internal audits on the implementation and effectiveness of all elements of the quality system in meeting stated aims of the service quality;

- changes due to new technologies, quality concepts, market strategies and social or environmental conditions.

The outcomes of such reviews should be included into management policy and strategies for the future operation of services.

Personnel and resources

The management should provide the necessary conditions and opportunities for the implementation of a quality system based on the stated aims and objectives embodied in a quality policy statement. These should include the needs of the personnel as well as the resources required for the provision of services.

Motivation

Creating structures and empowering personnel to participate in the QMS is not enough. Success also depends on motivating personnel so that they want to take on the responsibilities associated with QMS.

The achievement of this depends on taking into account a further development, generally known as *'quality management'*, which has been translated from its initial application in industrial production into service areas. This has been extended to the idea of total quality management (TQM) which has had a strong support from major industries. It has also a number of critics, especially as far as TQM in smaller enterprises is concerned.

Whether the issue is QMS or TQM, management needs to concentrate on the motivation, development, communication and performance of personnel, as follows:

- select personnel on the basis of competence to satisfy the job description;
- provide a work environment that fosters excellence and a secure job relationship;
- realise the potential of every employee by consistent, creative work methods and opportunities for greater involvement;
- see that all personnel feel that they have an involvement and influence on the quality of service provided to the customer;
- encourage contributions which enhance quality by giving due recognition and reward for achievement;
- periodically assess the factors which motivate the employees to provide quality service;
- implement career planning and development of personnel;
- establish planned actions for updating the competence and skills of the personnel.

Training and development

Education brings awareness of the need for change and provides the means of implementing it. The training elements include:

- training activities in quality management, including quality-related cost, and evaluation of the effectiveness of the QMS;
- training of personnel, which should not be limited only to those directly responsible for QMS;
- education of personnel about the organization's quality policy, objectives and specifications for satisfaction of patients' needs;
- a quality-awareness programme, which may include instructions and training courses for new entrants, as well as refresher courses for others;
- procedures for specifying and verifying that personnel have received suitable training;
- training in process control, data collection and analysis, problem identification and analysis, corrective action and improvement, team work and communication methods;
- the need to assess personnel requirements for formal qualifications and giving appropriate encouragement and support;
- the performance evaluation of personnel to assess their needs for development and potential.

Communication

The service personnel in direct or indirect contact with customers (i.e. patients and their families) should have the communication knowledge and skills necessary to be able to provide a high quality of service. They should also be able to work as a part of a team within the organization and be able to interact with other external organizations in the course of providing quality service to their customers.

A QMS depends on different groups of personnel with specific duties requiring the competence of the members in team work. A group can take the form of a quality improvement forum or quality circle, and members aim to improve quality of services by joint participation in the problem-solving processes.

Communication includes interaction within the management, between the management and employees, as well as among the employees. This can be enhanced through an effective information system and can include the following methods:

- management briefings;
- information exchange meetings;
- documented information;
- information technology facilities.

Material resources

The material required for the delivery of services may include:

- service provisioning equipment and stores;
- operational needs such as accommodation, transport, and information systems;
- quality-assessment facilities, instrumentation and computer facilities (hardware and software);
- operational and technical documentation.

Method of assessment

Evaluation of an activity related to the provision of services, based on the concept of quality, needs certain preparations. This is especially true of health promotion and health education services, which have so far no generally agreed specifications and procedures, since there has been little evaluation in this area and the few instruments that exist have been concerned with the measurement largely of efforts and outcomes.

The organizational model of health promotion and health education based on a settings approach includes a great variety of different settings (i.e. school, hospital, family, etc.), which require the development of specifications and procedures for each individually, since there are few health promotion and health education specifications and procedures already available.

The development of specifications is closely related to the aims of the organization or the intervention within an organization. These aims will need to be differentiated on the following levels:

- organizational level - this will include the aims of the organization in general as well as for its overall health promotional activities;
- process level - this will include the aims of the health promotion intervention;
- outcome level - this will define what kind of results are expected from the intervention.

The development of specifications for these three levels needs to reflect the relationship between them and the factors involved in evaluation, such as:

- aims - denote what is intended to be achieved;
- objectives - denote how it will be achieved;
- indicators - denote what will be used to assess the achievement;
- specifications - denote the acceptable level of quality and type of product;
- standards - denote the requirements for quality management.

Specifications

It is usual for specifications for the delivery of a service to be set by those in charge of defining such services and/or the professional bodies that are responsible for the activities of the staff providing the services. The approach to quality assessment is very similar to the established methods of evaluation in general. This will include the following steps:

Aims and objectives

The health promotion and health education intervention as a service provided by a setting needs clearly to define aims in order to be able to assess the outcomes. These aims should be closely linked to the achievement of standards and will represent the set specifications. The aims will have to be identified on three levels:

- the organizational level;
- the process level;
- the outcome level.

Once these aims have been defined, the next step is to define the objectives, which will reflect the ways these aims are to be achieved. Each of the aims may have several objectives. These objectives will represent the recognised procedures for the achievement of a specific aim and will include standard practices.

Indicators

The next step will be to choose which indicators will be used to assess the achievement of the aims. They will also be used to assess the relationship between the aims and objectives selected, or in quality terms, between specifications and procedures or standard practices.

To be able to draw any conclusions from the achievements as measured, they will have to be based on pre-set criteria which indicate what is and is not acceptable. This will show whether the achieved outcomes meet the set specifications and whether they can be defined in terms of whether a perceptible optimal and minimal outcome or a lack of any noticeable change for better or for worse.

Data collection

Aims and indicators need to be translated into instruments, which will be used to monitor the processes and outcomes. These instruments can be in the form of existing records, specially designed questionnaires, aide memoires for case studies or other tools for diagnosis and screening procedures.

Developing new QMS for HP/HE

There have been further developments in relating quality management to HP/HE, and in using it as a method of continuous evaluation of HP/HE activities within a Health Promoting Setting. Within an organizational framework, HP/HE can be considered as a part of the service industries and, owing to its specific character, it will require appropriate standards and specifications which could lead to its own certification system.

TQM AND HP/HE

Total Quality Management (TQM) has largely been developed to control production and, therefore, concentrates on this process. The production process as a whole is sub-divided into various input/output points in the system and each of these points is differentiated in terms of 'raw material' (RM) and 'end product' (EP).

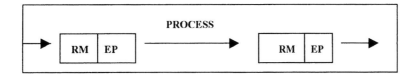

The first assumption of TQM is that any production process can be thus sub-divided into various production units. For example, a doctor-patient interaction in a general practitioner's surgery could be sub-divided into the following units: the family from which the patient comes, the receptionist as the first contact of the patient with the health care system, seeing the doctor, and then returning into the family and community. Each of these units in the system can be conceptualized as treating the patient as 'raw material' when he/she enters the unit and as the 'end product' when exiting from that unit. Of course, this does not imply that doctors would treat people in this depersonalised manner. It is just for purposes of conceptualising the overall system. It can be represented in a diagram.

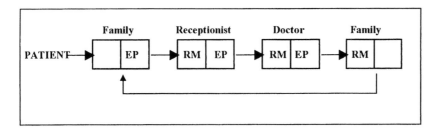

The diagram defines the points in the system in terms of functions, interactions and activities. At each of these points it is possible to differentiate the 'raw material - end product' aspects of the process: the patient leaves the family as its 'end product' and brings with him/her attitudes, habits, competencies and expectations acquired from the family into the process of assessing the meaning of a symptom; the patient enters the process of interaction with the health care system as 'raw material' and is treated as RM and EP in each of the steps in the process; when the receptionist receives the patient, he/she become her 'raw material' and after dealing with him/her in terms of exploratory talks, consulting records and making an appointment, the patient becomes the receptionist's 'end product' and receives an appointment to see the doctor; the doctor deals with the patient as 'raw material' through interview, examination, diagnosis and prescription of treatment and hands him/her over to the family as his 'end product'; the family receives the patient as its 'raw material' and the patient then undergoes the process of readjustment (or rehabilitation) to end as family's 'end product'. In this way the doctor-patient interaction is represented as a complex system including a number of factors as shown in the diagram.

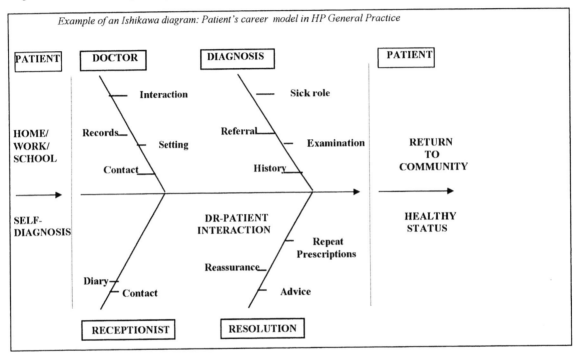

Example of an Ishikawa diagram: Patient's career model in HP General Practice

The various activities of each of these units provide a good basis for the quality assessment of the parts of the whole process. The patient moving between the described units of the system becomes exposed to a number of interaction activities, in all of which he/she is an active participant.

Using the 'raw material - end product' concept for each step of this interaction makes it possible for each actor to check the state of the 'raw material' received and thus ensure that the interaction has met the expected specifications by using agreed upon indicators and criteria. This is the most important concept involved in TQM, which defines the role of each actor in assessing the state or condition of the received raw material before processing it and handing it on as the end product of that interaction. When this is repeated throughout the whole process, any mistake can be corrected on the spot where it has been noticed. The rule of a TQM process is that there should be no failures in the output since all the corrections are made as a part of the production process.

The process and aspect of the quality assessment procedure has an advantage over traditional evaluation, which usually provides information about the success or failure of an intervention at the end of a whole process. There have been attempts to introduce 'process evaluation', but without formally recognized feedback mechanisms this can not ensure the quality of the outcome.

Greater detail in the description of the whole process in the example of a doctor-patient interaction illustrates this point. In the case of the doctor - patient example, the receptionist will be the first to assess the 'raw material' received from the family. If he/she notices that, for example, the patient lacks information about the operations of the general practice, he/she may remedy this by providing additional information to the patient. The doctor will assess the 'end product' of the receptionist, which now becomes the doctor's 'raw material'. If the doctor notices the receptionist's 'end product' is 'faulty' i.e. the patient has not been properly prepared for the oncoming meeting with the doctor, then the doctor will have to compensate for this omission by additional preparations of the patient or by referring the patient back to the receptionist. During the process of interaction (contact, history, examination, diagnosis, treatment) this 'raw material' becomes transformed into the doctor's 'end product' which is returned to the family. Now the family will assess the doctor's 'end product' in terms of defined specifications and treat the patient as their 'raw material'. If the family notices that the doctor's 'end product' does not meet the specifications, as for example, in the case when no preparations have been made for family support (resources, skills), the family will have a possibility to lodge a complaint to the proper authority and demand rectification of the omission.

DOCTOR - PATIENT INTERACTION				
FAMILY (EP)	PATIENT (RM/EP)	RECEPTIONIST (RM/EP)	DR (RM/EP)	FAMILY (RM)
Values	Competence	Setting	Setting	Social support
Structure	Status	Records	Records	Skills
Roles	Personality	Diary	History	
	Symptoms		Diagnosis	
	Compliance		Treatment	
LEGIT-IMIS-ATION	SYMPTOMS DECISION	APPOINT-MENT	DIAGNOSIS TREATMENT MONITORING	LEGIT-IMIS-ATION
WELL ROLE ⟶		SICK ROLE ⟶		WELL ROLE

* EP=end product; RM=raw material

For some production processes and services there are set standards, which are formalised and included in, the standards set by recognised organizations or institutions. One of these, *The British Standards Institution*, Handbook 22 "Quality Assurance" (described in Bendell et al. 1993, Munro-Faure et al. 1993) provide a whole set of standards, such as:

- BS 4778: Quality Vocabulary
- BS 4891: A Guide to Quality Assurance
- BS 5233: Glossary of Terms used in Metrology.
- BS 5750: Quality Systems
- BS 5760: Reliability of Constructed or Manufactured Products, Systems, Equipment and Components
- BS 5781: Measurement and Calibration Systems
- BS 6143: Guide to Economics of Quality
- BS 7000: Guide to Managing Product Design
- BS 7229: Guide to Systems Quality Auditing

In the course of time, standards are revised and replaced. For example, BS 5750 is no longer current.

The QMS for Health Promotion and Health Education

The introduction of a quality management system (QMS) for the specific purpose of assessing HP/HE activities within a setting needs to be developed as the extension of the combination of assessment, evaluation and auditing (see diagram page 160). The introduction of QMS for HP/HE will require a structure for the development of standards and specifications, a structure for accreditation and a supporting structure of consultants who will be able to help various settings to achieve the necessary transformation and meet the required standards for certification.

The previous section under the heading Certification, discusses the various requirements for the introduction of a QMS which could serve as a basis for the development of a specific HP/HE quality management system.

The organizational structures required can be illustrated in the following diagram:

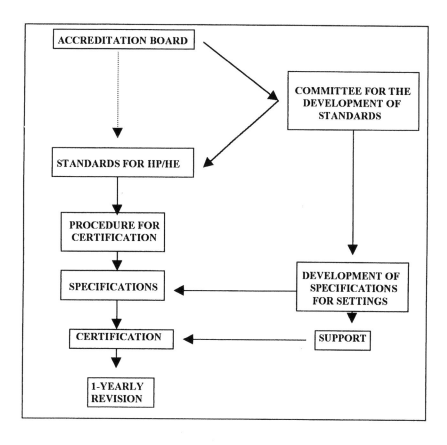

The development will need to include an *Accreditation Board*, under the chairmanship of an expert both in HP/HE and quality systems, and members who should represent both aspects of these activities. During the initial stage of the development of such a system it is necessary to have a *Committee* dealing with the development of standards and procedures for certification. Once the standards and the procedure have been agreed upon, the committee will have to develop specifications for each type of settings according to the needs of the stakeholders, staff and consumers. During the process of applying for certification, various settings will need support from *external experts* and consultants, approved by the Accreditation Board. The accredited settings need to be reviewed each year to ensure that the quality management is a continuous process within a setting.

The assessment of quality of HP/HE services, based on shared standards and specifications, has many advantages:

- It should unify the various HP/HE approaches and avoid those which are unsuccessful in terms of effectiveness, efficiency and customer satisfaction, including their health gain.

- This approach will be highly appropriate for 'Health Promoting Settings'. At present such settings need to belong to a national and international network and acquire recognition as a 'Health Promoting Setting' from the management of their network. During the experimental stage of the development of different 'Health Promoting Settings' such as schools, hospitals, etc., the management of the relevant networks has been limiting the number of settings for experimental reasons. The outcome was that each network consisted of 10 – 20 'pilot health promoting settings' with a recognized special status, which were allowed to use a WHO logo and acquire a competitive edge compared with other settings of the same kind in that country. This created conflicts within networks because of the exclusion of some settings, which were prepared to undertake similar commitment and were not admitted during the first phase of the project. By changing the system of accreditation to the certification of 'Health Promoting Settings', with quality management systems, it will remove such limitations and open the whole field to anyone who can meet the required standards and specifications;

- The introduction of QMS into Health Promoting Settings will use continuous quality assessment instead of the existing evaluation, which has suffered from so many problems and failures.

The need for a specific QMS for HP/HE is the logical outcome of the developments of a setting approach based on an organizational model. HP/HE are now a part of the service industry and should apply the same mechanisms for ensuring accountability as any other institution within that industry.

To find out what has happened after an intervention has taken place it will be necessary to measure the outcome. This measurement can have two aims:

- To find out whether the stated aims and objectives have been achieved (evaluation or evaluative audit), and
- To find out whether the achievements are in accordance with the existing social, professional, legal, cultural, religious, and other norms (audit proper).

Evaluation

Evaluation as related to HP/HE activities can be defined as the assessment *of the achievement of the stated aims of an intervention*. Although evaluation is only a part of the measuring accountability within a settings approach, it is appropriate for the measuring of the achievements of interventions within that setting.

Any evaluation will depend on the findings based on the data collected about the intervention and its outcome. To achieve credibility, the evaluation should meet the required level of scientific rigor in its methodology. The consumers of evaluation are the stakeholders; an effective evaluation receives recognition by contributing to action; and the aims of an evaluation are to allow a judgement to be made, by those involved, about the success or failure of an intervention.

The conceptualization of the research aspects of an evaluation depends on the precision in defining the **aims** and **objectives** of the intervention in measurable terms. The assumptions or hypotheses to be tested will depend on the set aims, and the effects of the intervention will depend on the relationship between the set aims and objectives and the resulting **outcomes**. The **methods** used in collecting data will depend on the scope of the intervention as well as on its aims and objectives. Depending on the aims, the collection of data can include hard or soft data. The size of the **population** will decide whether it will be necessary to carry out a sample survey or use a case study approach. The questions asked will depend on the choice of **indicators** intended to provide an insight into the area of inquiry. The kind of data involved will also define the most useful **instruments**. In case of a survey a questionnaire will be needed, whereas for a case study an aide-memoir may be necessary as a guide for an in-depth interview. The type of data collected will determine the applicable mode of **analysis**. In the case of a survey, a statistical analysis may be necessary, whereas different methods of analysis will be required for a qualitative analysis. The inferences will depend on the **criteria** agreed upon, which will help in deciding the level of achievement indicating success or failure. The outcome should also indicate any possible and unexpected side effects from the intervention.

```
┌─────────────────────────────────────────────────────────────────────┐
│                          EVALUATION                                    │
│                                                                        │
│   AIM 1......AIM n                                                      │
│                                                                        │
│        Objective 1.1.....Objective 1.n                                 │
│                                                                        │
│             Indicator 1.1.1......Indicator 1.1.n                       │
│                                                                        │
│                  Instrument 1.1.1.1.......Instrument 1.1.1.n           │
│                                                                        │
│                       Criteria 1.1.1.1.1.......Criteria 1.1.1.1.n      │
│                                                                        │
└─────────────────────────────────────────────────────────────────────┘
```

Once the **base line** has been established, the development of indicators and criteria, the collection of data and the inferences will follow the pattern defined by the requirements of recognized research methods. In this way the credibility of the findings will be enhanced.

There are various ways in which an evaluation can be carried out depending on what should be evaluated and how it should be done:

- *evaluation* in its broadest sense covers all procedures which allow a judgement about the success in achieving the stated aims of a project;

- *programme evaluation* provides a framework which covers all the aspects of a complex program, as in the case of a large scale activity in a hospital or a school;

- *project evaluation* deals with individual projects within a wider programme, as in the case of the required intervention studies within a health promoting hospital or school;

- *product evaluation* deals with the outcomes of programmes and projects, in terms of their products such as publications, materials or specific techniques, which can then be transferred to other similar settings and used in further interventions as well as for preparation of teaching material.

It will also be useful to differentiate evaluation according to the expectations associated with the outcome such as:

- *effectiveness,* which assesses the outcomes in terms of stated aims;

- *efficiency,* which aims to show that the objectives of the program are the best in terms of cost effectiveness and probability of achieving the desired outcome;

- *effort,* which aims to show whether a project is capital - or labour-intensive and gives an indication about the required resources necessary for a successful conclusion of a project or programme.

Since an evaluation will depend on the way the aims have been defined and the choice of appropriate objectives, it will be necessary to define these two concepts for the purposes of an evaluation programme:

- *aims* are defined as desired or planned outcomes of a programme or a project; they are usually stated in general terms and represent the basis for carrying out a project or a programme;

- *objectives* are defined as the means of achieving stated aims; an aim may have a number of different objectives which are related to the methods used as most appropriate for the achievement of the stated aims.

Sometimes planners understand quite different things when concepts are turned into actions. For evaluation, they need to state the aims precisely enough to be measured. They must also justify the choice of objectives for the achievement of each stated aim. This justification can be based on existing experience, empirical evidence or on tested theories. In some cases the objectives themselves may be the reason for evaluation. This can occur in situations where it is not clear which objectives can be linked to the achievement of aims and a set of alternative objectives may be tested as part of the evaluation project in order to discover those most appropriate. In this case, the evaluation process will be closely linked to the research processes related to the topic under study.

The decisions about aims and objectives can also be dependent on the interests of the stakeholders. Stakeholders are people who have a legitimate interest in the outcome of the project. If the evaluation does not take at least some of their needs into account, then it is hardly worth doing, since it will not make a contribution and is unlikely to be used. Usual stakeholders include: the staff carrying out a project; the consumers or clients of the project; the fund givers; or the management of the institution, which hosts the programme. In some cases evaluation is a part of a research project contracted from outside for the purpose of gaining information about the performance of the institution or the programme, or as a condition for the researchers gaining higher qualifications.

The aims and objectives will be decisive in choosing the most suitable type of evaluation methods, which can be:

- *monitoring* - this refers to keeping constant track of the progress of a project and can be a part of a more general evaluation;

- *assessment* - this is used to test the knowledge and skills of people involved in carrying out the objectives, as well as those considered to benefit from the outcomes;

- *appraisal* - this usually denotes a subjective assessment of a process which forms a part of the objectives; sometimes the term is applied to an evaluation of an individual's contribution as a whole;

- *formative evaluation* - this examines the process and the direction in which the programme or project is going with respect to the aims and objectives;

- *summative evaluation* - this examines the outcome and provides an insight into what has been done and whether it was worth doing in relation to the aims of the project or programme.

This differentiation of various kinds of evaluation is important, because it allows the evaluator to review the literature that deals with various aspects and provides detailed information about the methodology relevant to each type of evaluation.

The main methodological problem in evaluating a project is to choose the right *indicators* for the measurement of success or lack of it. The indicators will obviously be linked to aims but will also be relevant to the objectives chosen to achieve these aims. In a way it is a double measure: a sign of success or failure and a test of the links between aims and objectives. If the wrong objectives have been chosen for the achievement of an aim, then failure can be as much due to inappropriate objectives as to the wrong implementation of the right objectives. The evaluator should be reminded that an index may use variables or attributes, may distribute the findings on an ordinal or a cardinal scale, or may be expressed in a battery of questions, which jointly will represent an index or a scale. The indicators for the purpose of evaluation must be tested for *validity and reliability*. Validity implies that the instrument is measuring what it is supposed to measure, whereas reliability implies that a similar result will be obtained when other researchers repeat the same measurement.

Even when appropriate indicators have been chosen, the evaluator will be faced with the problem of deciding on the *criteria* that will indicate the success or failure of a project. The recognition of criteria relates to the acceptable levels expected to be achieved in a successful intervention and indicates the area of failure. In simple terms, 25% of positive replies in one study may be defined as success (for example in reduction of smoking), whereas in another study it may indicate a failure (as in an immunization programme). To identify the accepted level as a criterion of success it will often be necessary to consult specialists in the field, such as for example, doctors, teachers and other stakeholders.

The evaluation of the complex processes that are usually involved in a health promotion and health education intervention may require a multi-methodology approach, which will include a combination of a number of different instruments.

The evaluator should be aware that designing new instruments, as well as using some of the existing ones, requires expertise and in some cases, a recognized professional status, as is the case for example, with psychological tests.

Evaluative audit

There are situations where there is an obvious need for accountability and which would require an evaluation of a specific activity or programme, but where it is not possible because the programme in question does not have any defined aims and objectives on which an evaluation could be based. In such cases it is possible to carry out a special variety of evaluation known as 'shadow evaluation' (Rossi & Freeman, 1993) in which aims and objectives are assured. Another means of meeting the need for accountability is by evaluative auditing, which can be defined as *the assessment of a programme against some generally agreed upon specifications and using indicators and criteria relevant to these agreed expectations.*

Evaluative auditing applies the same approach as general evaluation with a number of specific modifications. It is possible, for the sake of convenience, to distinguish a number of distinctive stages in evaluative auditing, although in some cases the stages can become merged.

Aims and objectives

Where a programme or activity does not have any explicit aims, and for that reason an evaluative audit is being used, the aims will have to be set by the evaluator. If existing expectations are used, then an ordinary audit is possible, but if an attempt is made to assess the actions and programmes of health promotion and health education, going beyond these stated parameters, the evaluative audit will have define the 'expected aims'. These can then be used as the basis for evaluative audit.

The same process will apply to the definition of objectives. These can be assumed from the examination of the programme activities and related to the aims.

Once the aims and objectives have been identified, then it will be easy to select the appropriate indicators and agree about the acceptable criteria for the establishment of positive or negative outcomes.

Method

An evaluative audit will depend on the methods used to establish the existing expectations in terms of aims. This can be achieved *internally* by analyzing the objectives (activities, programmes) existing in the setting and deriving the assumed aims, which should reflect the reasons for the objectives.

Another way of establishing aims 'after the event' is to survey the various stakeholders. These can be subdivided into groups of individuals with common knowledge or expertise. The method of 'group interview' can then be used for each of the subgroups. There are several varieties of group interviews (Denzin & Lincoln, 1994) ranging from highly structured to free and unstructured ones:

- *focus group* interviews, which are formal and take place in a selected setting in which the role of the interviewer is directive and the questions are structured; such interviews are used for exploratory pre-test of instruments and situations;

- *nominal group* interviews, which are set in formal settings, in which the role of the interviewer is directive, questions are structured, and the use is exploratory or for pre-testing;

- *field (formal) group* interviews, which are set in prearranged and organized settings, but are carried out in the field, in which the role of the interviewer is somewhat directive, the questions are semi-structured, and it is used for descriptive and in-depth studies;

- *field (natural) group* interviews, which take place in informal or spontaneous settings, in which the role of the interviewer is moderately non-directive, the questions are very unstructured, and the use is for exploratory and ethnographic studies;

- *brainstorming*, which takes place in formal or informal settings, in which the role of the interviewer is non-directive, the questions are very unstructured, and it is used for exploratory purposes.

The method of group interviews will depend on the characteristics of the group members. To establish opinions about the possible aims within a setting, a number of groups may be involved, including:

- the group of *stakeholders* (authorities, professional organizations, grant giving bodies, etc.), who may provide the 'official' opinion about the expectations related to roles and the activities within a setting;

- the group of *experts or professionals* (the most knowledgeable people in the area, including professional experts such as teachers, doctors, other academics and specialists), who may provide a 'professional' opinion about the role and the activities of the setting;

- the group of *employees* (managers and workers), who may find themselves in the situation of defining in words what they are doing and why they are doing it in a particular way;

- the group of *consumers* (clients, patients, pupils, students, family members, etc.), who will be able to provide information about their interpretation of the setting is all about, what it is doing and what it could do in addition to improve their actions or programmes.

The interviewer needs to combine the skills of interviewing with the skills of running a group. The expertise required consists of the ability to listen, prompt and summarise individual statements and to be flexible, objective, emphatic, persuasive and a good listener; he/she should also have the skills to manage a group by preventing one person or a small coalition from dominating the group, encouraging reluctant members to participate, and to make sure to obtain the opinions of the whole group concerning the entire topic. The interviewer thus combines the role of the directive interviewer with the role of the group moderator. He/she must be simultaneously concerned with the questions and answers, as well as the processes of group dynamics.

To avoid the effects of group dynamics on the process and outcome a version of the *Delphi method* is often used (Scriven, 1991). This approach is based on the important role of the moderator who should be equal in expert knowledge to the respondents. The method of approach is to select groups of experts (stakeholders), but to avoid putting them in a face-to-face situation, thus avoiding irrelevant influence from group effects, where one person may sway a group's views. Instead, the mediator sends out a set of questions or statements and collects the answers from the respondents, asking them to provide the reasons for their choices. The mediator examines the answers, feeds them back to the group members with the respondents' explanations. This can be repeated several times until a consensus emerges. Each member has time without any external pressure to reconsider his/her statements. Such an approach is useful for obtaining expert opinions in deciding about the important points or in setting future trends of a programme. It has proved very effective in predicting change and in identifying solutions to problems.

In a group interview, discussions need to be continued until some agreement about the aims in the setting has been reached. This may require a number of meetings and good communications within the groups if the aims are to be shared and acted on.

Outcome

The outcome should be a consensus of opinions, within the groups involved in the exercise, about the aims of a programme or a setting. A possible way of keeping the group discussion on track is to relate the proposed aims to the existing objectives or activities within the setting. This should produce 'realistic' aims to be achieved by the effective objectives (or activities) pursued in the setting or in the programme. Another way of focusing the group's attention on the topic under discussion is to ask the members to illustrate the proposed aims, and link them with the indicators to be used in the measurement of such aims. Once the indicators have been agreed upon, the next step should be to reach an agreement on the criteria for success or failure. The outcome of the group activity should be the possibility of defining the aims, describing the objectives, selecting the indicators and reaching agreement on the criteria for an evaluative audit of a health promotion and health education activity as a special programme or as a part of a setting's activity.

Audit proper

The introduction of health promotion and health education activities into the auditing process, as well as the introduction of the auditing process into health promotion and health education activities is a relatively new idea. The former idea emerged when health promotion and health education activities switched from health problems, to people in settings with health problems, which brought about the need for a modification of health promotion and health education so that it was compatible with an organizational structure with its own system of evaluation, quality assessment and auditing. The latter idea became necessary as the demand for accountability of health promotion and health education activities grew and it was clear that many of them did not start by defining their aims and, therefore, could not be evaluated.

Auditing an activity or a setting can be defined *as the process of assessment against some external norm (legal, moral, religious, professional, etc.)*. The auditor usually has a recognized formal status and the auditee accepts the process of auditing as an integral part of the procedures of a setting or a programme.

Professional audit is concerned with settings or activities that are formalized and have institutionalized norms or expectations. There are situations where normal evaluation is not possible because the setting or the programme does not have set aims that would provide a basis for the evaluation. In such instances it is possible to assess the activities of a setting or a programme by using evaluative audit, which applies special methods of defining the aims 'after the event' and then carries out the process of assessment.

There are a number of activities, especially in the service industry, which depend on a 'provider - purchaser' interaction, in which the process as well as outcome have been externally defined. Although relevant settings have a built-in system of accounting, quality assessment and evaluation, they are also subject to auditing by specially designated bodies, which have a formally established responsibility for monitoring and assessing the process and the outcome of such services.

Financial audit

The best known example of a professional audit *is the assessment of the financial activities of a setting in terms of accuracy of recording and justification of disposing of the income and expenditure*. This type of audit has a long history originating in the 16th century when it was known as 'an official systematic examination of accounts' (Medicom, 1991). The 'aims and objectives' on which such an audit is based are usually defined in terms of an institution's plans concerning income and expenditure, or a budget, which is approved at the beginning of the financial year and which needs to be followed closely. The 'indicators and criteria' for such an audit are provided by laws and regulations concerning the finances and accounts of an institution. In this way both the auditor and the auditee are quite clear about the existing expectations and need only to follow them.

Even this straightforward system of auditing has recently been undergoing certain radical changes. In addition to using the usual indicators and criteria based on the legal norms related to laws and rules avoiding criminal activities and enshrined in a number of laws and regulations, there is now a new concept of 'green' audit. This adds to the usual indicators based on laws and regulations the idea of environmental protection. Organizations are now being audited for irregularities in handling the finances, as well as for the damaging effects their activities or products are having on the environment. In fact, auditing, like accounting, is subject to changes in practice, reflecting changing norms and values among the professionals involved.

Medical audit

Medical audit is an extension of the original concept of auditing. It is defined as *'the systematic critical analysis of quality of medical care.'* (Medicom, 1991). Medicom (1991) produced a Study Book on Medical Audit in their series of books on 'Teamwork'. The book is written in two parts, the first part including a self-assessment exercise with background information covering the topic under consideration and the second part including a group work module consisting of a video programme and discussion material. It is especially designed for general practices and provides an opportunity for each member of the practice to study it individually.

The description of the medical audit (Medicom, 1991) quotes Metcalfe, who suggested that everyone in medical audit will be looking for something different: the government and the FHSA would probably see audit as a means of ensuring good services for the money paid; general practitioners may use audit to ensure that what they think they are doing is close to what they are in fact doing; and managers will probably try to identify the top and the bottom of a range of quality of services so that they can persuade those at the bottom to improve their services.

Medical audit can be applied to three different activities: it may refer to the collection of information about an aspect of medical care and its presentation to colleagues, after which recommendations and comments about the standards of performance are made, which is also known as 'peer review'; or it may refer to the educational process which relates to the identification of a problem in health care delivery that can then be rectified; it may also refer to 'practice audit' which is mainly concerned with data collection used for reports as required by the Family Health Services Authority (FHSA).

Below is an example of how the issues have been explored in one FHSA (Salford, UK). In the course of discussion of the interpretation of the meaning and the aims of auditing of general practices, three levels of activity emerged:

Level 1 : This looks at what the practice is doing based on quantitative information, where examination of the data may indicate certain weak points in the system and can indicate where improvements are necessary;

Level 2 : This is concerned with the planning of change based on auditing clinical activities; this can be done with respect to a protocol or by just examining the activities in general; the outcome may be an improvement in clinical practice or an improvement in the protocol being used;

Level 3 : This is concerned with evaluating change and concentrates on an audit of critical or negative events occurring in a practice; it includes certain specified events, such as what preceded a maternal death, a child admission to hospital for asthma, etc; it explores the input prior to the event with the aim of deciding whether anything could have been improved at the time; this, however, does not cover auditing 'avoidable' events that may lead to future litigation.

The main reason for auditing is to improve the provision of services and to meet patients' expectations, as based for example on the DoH document *The Patient's Charter* (see Baric, 1994, Append 5.) Issues connected with auditing are of great importance at the time when GP contracts are discussed and revised, including GPs' commitments to auditing their practice and their activities.

The Medicom (1991) book refers to the 'audit cycle' as developed by Baker and Pressley ('The Practice Audit Plan'). The cycle includes three stages: deciding what should be happening; studying what is actually happening; and introducing necessary change. It is based on collecting the relevant data about *effort, efficiency and effectiveness* in the provision of care. The main characteristic is confidentiality concerning the data, with special reference to the need for reporting, which should not allow for identification of individual patients. Such an audit will require additional resources in terms of time and equipment. Economy of efforts can be achieved by role differentiation between the members of the practice, which should be based on the existing competence and skills of each member in data collection and analysis.

The introduction of the concept of a 'health promoting general practice' (Baric, 1994, pp. 347-394) will result in redefining many of the aspects of the existing medical audit including quality assessment. This quality assessment process needs to include the evaluation and auditing of the practice as a setting, the job satisfaction of the staff as well as the health gain of the patients. It should also include the links of the practice with other relevant institutions in the community for the purpose of providing continuous care of the patient.

Health promotion and health education audit

The reform of the NHS in the UK has resulted in a number of Department of Health documents, which have been concerned with the establishment of specifications related to the delivery of the health care.

The rights and duties defined in the 'Patient's Charter', mentioned above, as well as in the DoH document *The Health of the Nation* (Baric, 1994, Appendix 4), provide a basis for auditing health promotion and health education activities, by using as indicators the stated rights and duties of patients. Although so far there has not been a specific auditor designated to audit the performance of various health promotion officers and health promotion units, this possibility could arise as the result of an increased demand for accountability in health promotion services, corresponding to general accountability in the provision of health care.

The basis for auditing health promotion and health education activities in the present situation is provided by the wide range of professions and occupations, actively involved in providing health promotion and health education services. At present the concept of auditing health promotion and health education activities, without taking into account the settings in which they occur, is not sufficiently developed for application in practice. Therefore, most of the auditing of health promotion and health education activities will form a part of auditing the activities of the settings in which it takes place. For example, auditing health promotion and health education in general practice will need to form a part of auditing that general practice. It thus includes health promotion and health education indicators and criteria into the overall assessment of the general practice.

APPENDIX 1

THE JAKARTA DECLARATION
ON
LEADING HEALTH PROMOTION INTO THE 21ST CENTURY

Preamble

The Fourth International Conference on Health Promotion: New Players for a New Era - Leading Health Promotion into the 21st Century, meeting in Jakarta from 21 to 25 July 1997, has come at a critical moment in the development of international strategies for health. It is almost 20 years since the World Health Organization's Member States made an ambitious commitment to a global strategy for Health for All and the principles of primary health care through the Declaration of Alma Ata. It is 11 years since the First International Conference on Health Promotion was held in Ottawa, Canada. That Conference resulted in proclamation of the Ottawa Charter for Health Promotion, which has been a source of guidance and inspiration for health promotion since that time. Subsequent international conferences and meetings have further clarified the relevance and meaning of key strategies in health promotion, including healthy public policy (Adelaide, Auastralia, 1988), and supportive environments for health (Sundsvall, Sweden, 1991).

The Fourth International Conference on Health Promotion is the first to be held in a developing country, and the first, to involve the private sector in supporting health promotion. It has provided an opportunity to reflect on what has been learned about effective health promotion, to re-examine the determinants of health, and to identify the directions and strategies that must be adopted to address the challenges of promoting health in the 21st century.

The participants in the Jakarta Conference hereby present this Declaration on action for health promotion into the next century.

Health promotion is a key investment

Health is a basic human right and is essential for social and economic development. Increasingly, health promotion is being recognised as an essential element of health development. It is a process of enabling people to increase control over, and to improve, their health. Health promotion, through investment and action, has a marked impact on the determinants of health so as to create the greatest health gain for people, to contribute significantly to the reduction of inequalities in health, to further human rights, and to build social capital. The ultimate goal is to increase health expectancy, and to narrow the gap in health expectancy between countries and groups.

The Jakarta Declaration Health Promotion offers a vision and focus for health promotion into the next century. It reflects the firm commitment of participants in the Fourth International Conference On Health Promotion to draw upon the widest possible range of resources to tackle health determinants in the 21st century.

211

Determinants of health: new challenges

The prerequisites for health care peace, shelter, education, social security, social relations, food, income, the empowerment of women, a stable eco-system, sustainable resource use, social justice, respect for human rights, and equity. Above all, poverty is the greatest threat to health.

Demographic trends such as urbanization, an increase in the number of older people and the high prevalence of chronic diseases pose new problems in all countries. Other social, behavioural and biological changes such as increased sedentary behaviour, resistance to antibiotics and other commonly available drugs, increased drug abuse, and civil and domestic violence threaten the health and well-being of hundreds of millions of people.

New and re-emerging infectious diseases, and the greater recognition of mental health problems, require an urgent response. It is vital that approaches to health promotion evolve to meet changes in the determinants of health.

Transnational factors also have a significant impact on health. These include the integration of the global economy, financial markets and trade, wide access to media and communications technology, and environmental degradation as a result of the irresponsible use of resources.

These changes shape people's values, their lifestyles throughout the lifespan, and living conditions across the world. Some have great potential for health, such as the developments of communications technology, while others, such as international trade in tobacco, have a major negative impact.

Health promotion makes a difference

Research and case studies from around the world provide convincing evidence that health promotion is effective. Health promotion strategies can develop and change lifestyles, and have an impact on the social, economic and environmental conditions that determine health. Health promotion is a practical approach to achieving greater equity in health.

The five strategies se out in the Ottawa Charge for Health Promotion are essential for success:

- build healthy public policy
- create supportive environments
- strengthen community action
- develop personal skills
- reorient health services

There is now clear evidence that:

- comprehensive approaches to health development are the most effective. Those that use combinations of the five strategies are more effective than single track approaches;

- particular settings offer practical opportunities for the implementation of comprehensive strategies. These include mega-cities, islands, cities, municipalities, local communities, markets, schools, the workplace, and health care facilities;

- participation is essential to sustain efforts. People have to be at the centre of health promotion action and decision-making processes for them to be effective;

- health learning fosters participation. Access to education and information is essential to achieving effective participation and the empowerment of people and communities.

These strategies are core elements of health promotion and are relevant for all countries.

New responses are needed

To address emerging threats to health, new forms of action are needed. The challenge for the coming years will be to unlock the potential for health promotion inherent in many sectors of society, among local communities, and within families.

There is a clear need to break through traditional boundaries within government sectors, between governmental and non-governmental organizations, and between the public and private sectors. Cooperation is essential; this requires the creation of new partnerships for health, on an equal footing, between the different sectors at all levels of governance in societies.

Priorities for health promotion in the 21st Century

1. Promote social responsibility for health

Decision-makers must be firmly committed to social responsibility. Both the public and private sectors should promote health by pursuing policies and practices that:

- avoid harming the health of individuals
- protect the environment and ensure sustainable use of resources
- restrict production of and trade in inherently harmful goods and substances such as tobacco and armaments, as well as discourage unhealthy marketing practices
- safeguard both the citizen in the marketplace and the individual in the workplace
- include equity-focused health impact assessments as an integral part of policy development

2. Increase investments for health development

In many countries, current investment in health is inadequate and often ineffective. Increasing investment for health development requires a truly multisectoral approach including, for example, additional resources for education and housing as well as for the health sector. Greater investment for health and reorientation of existing investments, both within and among countries, has the potential to achieve significant advances in human development, health and quality of life.

Investments for health should reflect the needs of particular groups such as women, children, older people, and indigenous, poor and marginalized populations.

3. Consolidate and expand partnerships for health

Health promotion requires partnerships for health and social development between the different sectors at all levels of governance and society. Existing partnerships need to be strengthened and the potential for new partnerships must be explored.

Partnerships offer mutual benefit for health through the sharing of expertise, skills and resources. Each partnership must be transparent and accountable and be based on agreed ethical principles, mutual understanding and respect. WHO guidelines should be adhered to.

4. Increase community capacity and empower the individual

Health promotion is carried out *by* and *with* people, not *on* or *to* people. It improves both the ability of individuals to take action, and the capacity of groups, organizations or communities to influence the determinants of health.

Improving the capacity of communities for health promotion requires practical education, leadership training , and access to resources. Empowering individuals demands more consistent, reliable access to the decision-making process and the skills and knowledge essential to effect change.

Both traditional communication and the new information media support this process. Social, cultural and spiritual resources need to be harnessed in innovative ways.

5. Secure an infrastructure for health promotion

To secure an infrastructure for health promotion, new mechanisms for funding it locally, nationally and globally must be found. Incentives should be developed to influence the actions of governments, non-governmental organizations, educational institutions and the private sector to make sure that resource mobilization for health promotion is maximized.

'Settings for health' represent the organizational base of the infrastructure required for health promotion. New health challenges mean that new and diverse networks need to be created to achieve intersectoral collaboration. Such networks should provide mutual assistance within and among countries and facilitate exchange of information on which strategies have proved effective and in which settings.

Training in and practice of local leadership skills should be encouraged in order to support health promotion activities. Documentation of experiences in health promotion through research and project reporting should be enhanced to improve planning, implementation and evaluation.

All countries should develop the appropriate political, legal, educational , social and economic environments required to support health promotion.

Call for action

The participants in this Conference are committed to sharing the key messages of the Jakarta Declaration with their governments, institutions and communities, putting the actions proposed into practice, and reporting back to the Fifth International Conference on Health Promotion.

In order to speed progress towards global health promotion, the participants endorse the formation of a global health promotion alliance. The goal of this alliance is to advance the priorities for action in health promotion set out in this Declaration.

Priorities for the alliance include:

- raising awareness of the changing determinants of health
- supporting the development of collaboration and networks
- mobilizing resources for health promotion
- accumulating knowledge on best practice
- enabling shared learning
- promoting solidarity in action
- fostering transparency and public accountability in health promotion

National governments are called on to take the initiative in fostering and sponsoring networks for health promotion both within and among their countries.

The participants call on WHO to take the lead in building such a global health promotion alliance and enabling its Member States to implement the outcomes of the Conference. A key part of this role is for WHO to engage governments, non-governmental organizations, development banks, organizations of the United Nations system, interregional bodies, bilateral agencies, the labour movement and cooperatives, as well as the private sector in advancing the priorities for action in health promotion.

Baldwin, T.S., McVoy, D.S., Steinfield, C. (1996) **Convergence – Integrating Media, Information and Communication**, Sage Publications, London.

Baric, L. (1991) **Health Promotion and Health Education – Problems and Solutions, Module 1**, Barns Publications, Hale Barns, Cheshire, 2nd edition. 1991.

Baric, L. (1994) **Health Promotion and Health Education in Practice – The Organisational Model, Module 2,** Barns Publications, Hale Barns, Cheshire.

Baric, L., Baric, L.F., (1995a) **Health Promotion and Health Education: Evaluation, Quality, Audit, Module 3,** Barns Publications, Hale Barns, Cheshire.

Baric, L. (1995b) **Curricula for Courses and Workshops in Health Promotion and Health Education,** Barns Publications, Hale Barns, Cheshire.

Baric, L. (1996) **Health Promotion and Health Education – Handbook for Students and Practitioners**, Barns Publications, Hale Barns, Cheshire.

Becker, H.A., (1997) **Social Impact Assessment**, UCL Press, London.

Bendell, T., Kelly, J., Merry, T., & Sims, F. (1993) *Quality : Measuring and Monitoring*, The Sunday Times Business Skills, Century Business, London.

Berelson, B., & Steiner, G.A. (1964) **Human Behaviour : An Inventory of Scientific Findings**, Brace and World Inc. New York.

Blake, R.B., & Mouton, J.S. (1985) **The Managerial Grid III,** Gulf Publishing Co.

Brown, T.A., (1989) **Genetics – A Molecular Approach,** Van Nostrand Reinhold, London.

Burdge, R.J., (1994a) **A Community Guide to Social Impact Assessement**, Social Ecology Press, Middleton.

Burdge, R.J., (1994b) **A Conceptual Approach to Social Impact Assessment** : Collection of Writings by Rabel Burdge and colleagues, Social Ecology Press, Middleton.

Burdge, R.J., and Robertson, R.A., (1994) "Social Impact Assessment and the Public Involvement Process", *Environmental Impact Assessment Review*, Volume 10 (1/2) pp.81-90.

Canter, L.W., (1996) **Environmental Impact Assessment**, McGraw Hill, New York.

Cameron, K.S. (1984) "The Effectiveness of Ineffectiveness", in B.M. Staw and LL. Cummings, ed. *Research in Organizational Behaviour*, Vol.6, JAI Press, Greenwich, Conn.p.276.

Clark, J.V., & Krone, C.G. (1972) "Towards an Overall View of Organizational Development in the Early Seventies" in J.M. Thomas and W.G. Bennis (eds), **Management of Change and Conflict**, Penguin, Harmondsworth.

Coile, R.C., (1986) **The New Hospital : Future Strategies for a Changing Industry**, Aspen Publishers, Rockville, MD.

Dawson, S. (1992) Analysing Organisations, 2nd edn. Billing & Sons, Worcester.

Denzin, N.K., Lincoln, Y.S. (1994) *Handbook of Qualitative Research*, Sage Publications, London.

Derrida, J. (1976) **Speech and Phenomenon**, Northwestern University Press, Evanston, Iln.

Drucker, P.F. (1968) **The Practice of Management**, Pan Books, London

Ernst, M., Stroheim, G. (1997) *The Viennese TQM Project – An Example to Implement TQM in the Organization of Hospitals,* paper presented at the 4th European Conference of the International Union for Health Promotion and Education, 9-12 November 1997, Israel.

Evans, D., Head, M.J., Speller, V. (1994) *Assuring Quality in Health Promotion*, Health Education Authority, London.

Finsterbusch, K., and Wolf, C.P., (eds) (1981) **Methodology of Social Impact Assessment** second edition, Hutchinson Ross, Stroudsburg.

Foucault, M (1977) **Discipline and Punish**, Pantheon, New York.

Habermas, J. (1971) **Toward a Rational Society**, Heinemann, London.

Hammer, M., & Champy, J. (1993) **Reengineering the Corporation – A Manifesto for Business Revolution**, Nicholas Brealey Publishing, London.

Hunt, J. (1979) **Managing People at Work,** Pan Books, London.

Lauffer, A. (1982) *Assessment Tools,* Sage Publications, London.

Lewin, K. (1953) **A Dynamic Theory of Personality: Selected Papers,** Translated by Adams D.K., & Zener, K.E., McGraw Hill Book Co. Inc. New York.

Likert, R. (1961) **New Patterns of Management**, McGraw Hill, London.

March, J.G., & Simon, H. (1958) **Organizations**, John Wiley, New York.

Marcuse, H. (1964) **One-Dimensional Man**, Beacon Press, Boston, USA.

Mayo, E. (1945) **The Social Problems of an Industrial Civilization**, Graduate School of Business Administration, Harvard University, Boston.

McGregor, D. (1987) **The Human Side of Enterprise,** Penguin, London.

Medicom (1991) *Medical Audit*, Study Book, Teamwork Series, Medicom UK, Kingston-upon-Thames.

Milloy, S. (1995) **Science Without Sense – The Risky Business of Public Health Research,** Cato Institute, Washington DC.

Mitchell, T.R. (1982) "Motivation: New Directions for Theory, Research and Practice" *Academy of Management Review,* vol. 7. No.1, pp.80-88.

Mitchell, T.R., Larson, J.R. (1987) **People in Organizations,** McGraw Hill, New York.

Moi, T. (1985) **Sexual/texual Politics: Feminist Libterary Theory,** Methuen, New York.

Moreno, J.L. (1953) **Who Shall Survive?** Beacon House, New York.

Morgan, G. (1993) **Imaginization – The Art of Creative Management,** Sage Publications, London.

Mullins, L.J. (1992) **Management and Organizational Behaviour,** Pitman, London.

Munro-Faure, L., Munro-Faure, M., Bones, E. (1993) *Achieving Quality Standards,* Institute of Management, Pitman Publishing, London.

Langford, V. (1979) "Managerial Effectiveness : A Review of the Literature" in Brodie, M., & Bennet, R. (eds) **Perspectives of Managerial Effectiveness,** Thames Valley Regional Management Centre.

O'Doherty, E. (1997) *'Healthmark' – Implementing the International Quality Assurance Standard ISO 9000, to Raise Quality in Health Promotion Services,* paper presented at the 4th European Conference of the International Union for Health Promotion and Education, 9-12 November 1997, Israel.

Ouchi, W.G. (1984) **Theory Z : How American Business Can Meet the Japanese Challenge,** Addison Wesley.

Pascale, R.T. (1990) **Managing on the Edge: The Learning Organization,** Simon and Schuster, New York.

Peter L.J., and Hall R., (1969) **The Peter Principle: Why Things go Wrong.** Morrow, New York.

Pugh, D.S. (1991) "Foreword" in Huczynski, A., & Buchanan, D., **Organizational Behaviour,** Prentice Hall, Hemel Hempstead, Herts.

Reddin, W.J. (1970) **Managerial Effectiveness,** McGraw Hill, London.

Robbins, S.P. (1990) **Organization Theory : Structure, Design and Applications,** 3rd edn. Prentice Hall International, Inc. London.

Rogers, R.W. (1975) "A Protection Motivation Theory of Fear Appeals and Attitude Change" in *Journal of Psychology* 91, (pp.93-114).

Rossi, P.H. & Freeman, H.E. (1985) *Evaluation: a Systematic Approach* (3rd edn), Sage Publications, London.

Schien, E.H. (1985) "Organizational Culture" in *Organizational Dynamics*, Vol. 12. pp.13-28.

Scriven, M. (1991) Evaluation Thesaurus (4th edn), Sage Publications, London.

Taylor, C.N., Bryan, C.H., and Goodrich, C.G., (1990) **Social Assessment : Theory, Process and Techniques**, second edition, Taylor Baines Associates, Lincoln.

Tse, KK. (1985) **Marks and Spencer**, Pergamon Press, London.

Twomey, J., and Tomkins, J.M., (1993) "Evaluation of Health Promotion", *Project Appraisal*, Volume 8 (1), pp.23-31.

WHO (1978) **The Alma Ata Declaration** in Alma Ata 1978 Primary Health Care, Geneva, WHO 1978 "Health for All" series No.1.

WHO (1984) **Targets for Health for All**, WHO, Geneva.

WHO (1986) **The Ottawa Charter for Health Promotion** in Health Promotion No.1, 1986, iii-v.

WHO (1988) **The Adelaide Recommendations: Healthy Public Policy** in Health Promotion 3 (2) 183-186, 1988.

WHO, CE , CEC (1993a) **The European Network of Health Promoting Schools**, WHO EURO, Copenhagen, 1993, (EUR/HPS3).
WHO (1993b) **Health Promotion in the Work Setting**, jointly with the Federal Centre for Health Education, Cologne, Germany, Verlag fur Gesundheitsforderung, G. Conrad, Gamburg, 1993.

WHO (1997) **The Jakarta Declaration "New Players for a New Era – Leading Health Promotion into the 21st Century"**, WHO, Geneva, 1997.